Endorsements

A blow by blow account by the key players in NCID, MOH and related agencies to apply the lessons learnt from SARS. A must read for all those with an interest in public health and infectious diseases in Singapore. This tome showcases the historical epic effort of many. Documenting it in the midst of the pandemic in itself is a herculean task. Kudos to the authors and the key actors for pulling such a feat.

Clinical Associate Professor Tan Thuan Tong,
Senior Consultant & Head, Department of Infectious Diseases,
Singapore General Hospital

This is an important and insightful capture of the multi-sectoral partnerships, as well as the planning and preparations that Singapore put in both before and during the COVID-19 outbreak, that allowed Singapore to respond effectively to manage the exceptional public health crisis.

Professor Teo Yik Ying,
Dean, Saw Swee Hock School of Public Health,
National University of Singapore

COVID-19 has brought home cogently the point that unilateral actions have little chance of success and that we must pull together to overcome this pandemic. Besides showcasing the remarkable knowledge we have gleaned in the short time since SARS-CoV-2 arrived on our shores, this book reflects nicely the collective and coordinated efforts that Singapore has taken along with our international partners to combat COVID-19.

Professor Chong Yap Seng,
Lien Ying Chow Professor in Medicine & Dean,
NUS Yong Loo Lin School of Medicine

Singapore has mounted a sophisticated, comprehensive and successful response to the spread of the COVID-19 virus, with remarkably low loss of life. This compendium of stories places the pivotal contribution of NCID in the context of Singapore's and the world's struggle to survive the pandemic. I am greatly impressed by the very rapid co-ordination of such a complex campaign, involving public health, laboratory, clinical and research modalities. What strikes me in all these reports, particularly the personal stories, is a wonderfully high level of morale, mutual trust and confidence in a positive outcome. This attitude is undoubtedly underpinned by a high level of preparedness and outstanding leadership and teamwork. It is an inspiring and compelling account from Singapore of the 2020 pandemic that has shaken the world.

Professor James Best,
Visiting Professor and Former Dean,
Lee Kong Chian School of Medicine

Working closely together, researchers and clinicians from Duke-NUS and NCID demonstrated the full value of multi-disciplinary research moving from bedside-to-bench and back. As this book chronicles, these teams advanced understanding of this novel coronavirus and its origins, including significant breakthroughs in serological testing. Their contributions emerged as the first COVID-19 cases appeared in Singapore, while the rest of the world was just coming to grips with the magnitude of the pandemic. Collaborations like this transform medicine and improve lives.

Professor Thomas Coffman,
Dean,
Duke-NUS Medical School

The COVID-19 pandemic is unfolding as the greatest crisis of our age. Having mounted a valiant response to keep the virus at bay, Singapore has emerged from the initial phase of the pandemic undefeated and unbowed, with our heads held high. This book chronicles the heroic efforts of public agencies, healthcare institutions, academia and ordinary Singaporeans in these initial months, including the leading roles NCID played. It contains valuable lessons on the importance of decisive leadership combined with an evidence-based, collaborative and whole-of-society approach in pandemic response.

Professor Yeoh Khay Guan,
Chief Executive,
National University Health System

2020 will always be etched in history as the year a pandemic brought the world to its knees and disrupted everybody's life, without exception. Singapore was no different from the rest of the world in that we were not expecting such an unprecedented massive disruption from a novel virus. However we were fortunate on many counts, like having battled SARS in 2003, to be more prepared to tackle the many unknowns in this crisis. Four months before the first patient was diagnosed in Singapore, the National Centre for Infectious Diseases (NCID) was officially launched. The NCID played a leading role in the successes that we have had.

This book is an excellent read that is written with clarity and precision. The authors give first person accounts of the various aspects of this defining period and there are many learning points that are well documented.

I would highly recommend this book to both healthcare professionals and the general public.

Professor Ivy Ng,
Group Chief Executive Officer,
Singapore Health Services Pte Ltd

COVID-19 has changed the world. NCID has been at the forefront of Singapore's fight against COVID-19 and has rallied the research community to make a real difference in the global COVID-19 battle. I congratulate Yee Sin, Paul and the many eminent authors who have contributed to this book, which will serve as a record of this "crisis of a generation" for many generations to come.

Associate Professor Tan Say Beng,
Executive Director,
National Medical Research Council

This book provides a thorough overview of the COVID-19 outbreak and management response to the pandemic in Singapore. It is very well written with fascinating personal stories. We are fortunate that we have great leaders in healthcare in Singapore including many in Infectious Diseases, who helped tackle the problem with a pragmatic approach, from planning ahead, curbing community transmission by implementing stepwise social distancing measures and carefully balancing public health demands with the country's economy. We can learn so much from the valuable insights provided — congratulations on this outstanding publication!

Professor Aung Tin,
Chief Executive Officer, Singapore National Eye Centre;
Senior Consultant, Glaucoma Dept, Singapore National Eye Centre;
Chair, Ophthalmology & Visual Sciences Academic Clinical Program,
Duke-NUS Medical School;
Kwan Im Thong Hood Cho Temple Professor of Ophthalmology,
Duke-NUS Medical School;
Associate Dean, Office of Research, Duke-NUS Medical School;
Group Director, Research (Scientific), SingHealth

Every pandemic is different. Different lessons, both positive and negative, can be drawn to prepare not just the health system but the whole country for the next pandemic. The next pandemic will come and it may be the dreaded Disease X, with high person to person transmission as well as high case fatality rates. Countries will need to take a comprehensive and organised systems approach to analyse their response to COVID-19 so that they will be prepared for Disease X. The starting point is proper documentation.

This book is an excellent record of the COVID-19 pandemic, seen through the eyes of Singapore's frontline personnel: from doctors to nurses, policy analysts and policymakers, medical technologists, researchers and modellers and public health specialists. It highlights the areas where we have done well: the well-coordinated whole-of-government approach with strong input from the academic and healthcare community. It also does not shy away from topics which the lay public perceived as less than perfect in the handling of the crisis like the massive third wave of the outbreak among dormitory migrant workers or the change in mask wearing advisories.

The book also highlights the very low fatality rate and very low infection rates among healthcare professionals. These are very crucial outcome indicators for any country managing this pandemic, especially when there is a strong temptation to focus on output indicators like the number of cases. The authors have attempted to suggest the factors that contributed to these outcomes: however a more formal system-level analysis will be needed in the future including the impact of the pandemic on the mortality and morbidity rates of non-COVID cases.

The personal stories from doctors, nurses, allied health staff and porters were a joy to read. It was refreshing and speaks of their commitment, dedication and resilience in the midst of fear and uncertainty. These give a human face to the concept of pandemic preparedness.

Professor Chia Kee Seng,
Professor, Saw Swee Hock School of Public Health,
National University of Singapore and
Professor, Yong Loo Lin School of Medicine,
National University of Singapore

Thoughtful, scholarly, thorough. COVID-19 Pandemic in Singapore is a must-read primer for those wanting to understand the SARS-CoV-2 phenomenon — it spans from virology, COVID-19's global spread, the early response in Singapore and worldwide, to shared experiences from those on the pandemic's front-line. The many authors' expertise is evidenced in their chronicling the rigorous planning and action taken to tackle the public health needs of Singapore's different populations, diagnostics, clinical management, infrastructure expansion, manpower deployment, community engagement, and clinical research needed to mount a campaign which has thus far been successful. I highly recommend COVID-19 Pandemic in Singapore.

Associate Professor David Allen,
Associate Vice President (Health Innovation and Translation),
National University of Singapore;
Associate Professor, Yong Loo Lin School of Medicine,
National University of Singapore

Healthcare is always in between outbreaks and our response always a work-in-progress as we learn with every outbreak. No outbreak is ever the same but the people we have and the relationships we build ready us for the next one. I am incredibly proud of my colleagues who have stood as the first and last line of defence against the COVID-19 pandemic.

Adjunct Professor Eugene Fidelis Soh,
Chief Executive Officer,
Tan Tock Seng Hospital and Central Health,
National Healthcare Group

This is a book about a country that was prepared for the pandemic of COVID-19 because it had applied lessons from previous responses to SARS, pandemic influenza, and Zika; and more exotic diseases such as human monkeypox. It is an important case study, written by experts in Singapore, of how one country dealt with the COVID-19 pandemic from the detection of first infections to gaining epidemiological and clinical understanding, and then using this to implement evidence-based measures that made Singapore's response exemplary, including its concept of a "circuit breaker". The testimonies of medical workers in the last chapter are especially poignant and describe their emotions, concerns, and devotion.

Professor David L. Heymann,
Professor of Infectious Disease Epidemiology,
London School of Hygiene & Tropical Medicine

This book highlights the significant contributions by Singaporean colleagues toward successful control of the COVID-19 pandemic in Singapore, and shows what can be achieved through coordinated, collaborative, and integrated partnerships among public health epidemiologists, clinicians, clinical investigators, and laboratory scientists to effectively respond to emerging infectious disease threats.

Dr Tim Uyeki,
Centers for Disease Control and Prevention,
Atlanta, Georgia

While the world still battles the COVID-19 pandemic, this book provides a useful and comprehensive synthesis of country case studies, disease epidemiology, and the containment measures and actions taken by Singapore to control the spread of the virus. It shows clear insight into the hurdles and successes of the Singapore response, providing lessons learnt which could and should be used by other nations. The opportunity to learn from the expertise and experience of colleagues in Singapore has been a longstanding privilege. The book will also be valuable in planning for future pandemics and in outbreak responses.

Professor Alison Holmes,
Professor of Infectious Diseases, Imperial College London and
President of the International Society for Infectious Diseases

As of November 15, 2021, the COVID-19 pandemic has caused more than 250 million infections and more than 5 million deaths worldwide. Singapore was forward-thinking in creating and building a National Centre for Infectious Diseases following SARS in 2003 and the H1N1 influenza pandemic in 2009. The Centre was designed to respond to the emergence of a new pathogen and SARS-CoV-2 was exactly that. In this book, scientists, clinicians, epidemiologists, including academics and policy makers from Singapore have written about their experiences and response to the COVID-19 pandemic. As 2021 draws to a close, 7 billion doses of vaccine have been administered, but the vaccine uptake has not been uniform throughout the world; millions of people are still suffering and many countries are struggling with waves of COVID-19. The global public health, medical and scientific community must learn from each other. This book, that narrates the Singapore experience is very timely, informative and inspiring. I congratulate the authors for sharing their insights in these challenging times.

Professor Kanta Subbarao,
Director, WHO Collaborating Centre for Reference and Research
on Influenza and Department of Microbiology and Immunology
at the Peter Doherty Institute for Infection and Immunity,
Melbourne, Australia

COVID-19 Pandemic Singapore in

COVID-19 Pandemic Singapore in

Editors

Leo Yee-Sin

National Centre for Infectious Diseases, Singapore

Paul Tambyah

National University of Singapore, Singapore

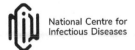
National Centre for
Infectious Diseases

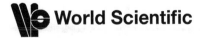
World Scientific

Published by

World Scientific Publishing Co. Pte. Ltd.

5 Toh Tuck Link, Singapore 596224

USA office: 27 Warren Street, Suite 401-402, Hackensack, NJ 07601

UK office: 57 Shelton Street, Covent Garden, London WC2H 9HE

British Library Cataloguing-in-Publication Data

A catalogue record for this book is available from the British Library.

COVID-19 PANDEMIC IN SINGAPORE

ISBN 978-981-123-937-3 (hardcover)
ISBN 978-981-123-982-3 (paperback)
ISBN 978-981-123-938-0 (ebook for institutions)
ISBN 978-981-123-939-7 (ebook for individuals)

For any available supplementary material, please visit
https://www.worldscientific.com/worldscibooks/10.1142/12344#t=suppl

Contents

Foreword

by Associate Professor Kenneth Mak
Director of Medical Services, Ministry of Health

2020 and 2021 were two of the most challenging years in recent memory. Not many would have predicted that an influenza-like virus would cause such a massive and prolonged disruption globally — cross-border travel has drastically declined, businesses have been forced to shut down, social gatherings are discouraged, and working from home has become the new way of life.

Singapore has also keenly felt the impact of the COVID-19 pandemic. The Multi-Ministry Taskforce was set up to coordinate a whole-of-government response to the COVID-19 outbreak, putting in place travel restrictions to stop the virus transmission to our shores, creating assistance packages to support those in need, and developing safe management measures to prevent viral transmission in the community. The pandemic has pushed us, as a society, to adapt to changes in the way we live, work and interact.

Despite these trying times, we have witnessed many acts that reaffirm the strength and grit of our people. Singaporeans were also proactive in our fight against COVID-19. Singaporeans from all walks of life stepped up to serve the nation: retired nurses returned to take up jobs in the healthcare sector, public sector officers offered their time to assist with contact tracing and other operational tasks, and volunteers rallied together to distribute essentials to fellow Singaporeans. In the community, Singaporeans, young and old, adapted to public health measures with great fortitude. Everyone made sacrifices, big and small — indeed, it has been a whole-of-society effort.

This book, put together by the National Centre for Infectious Diseases, captures the spirit of collaboration as various authors and sectors provide an account of the responses to the outbreak in Singapore. I am happy to have witnessed how our healthcare sector had harnessed the experience from past outbreaks, and how the sectors worked hand in hand at the frontline of this COVID-19 pandemic in the past two years.

Even as we adjust our measures progressively for a safe reopening, we must remember that the fight is not over. Many countries are facing second, third and fourth waves of the virus and continue to implement various measures against the pandemic. Singapore cannot be complacent. We must continue to stand in solidarity in this herculean effort against COVID-19.

Foreword

by Professor Philip Choo

Group Chief Executive Officer, National Healthcare Group

In January 2020, the world was faced with a new and unknown emerging infectious disease. What we now know as COVID-19 started in Wuhan, China and quickly spread across the globe. The World Health Organization announced it as a pandemic in just a few short months on 11 March 2020. Singapore was not spared and our first case was diagnosed on 23 January 2020. There are now millions of individuals worldwide who have been infected and more than six million associated deaths.

It was fortunate that the National Centre for Infectious Diseases (NCID) was built in time and officially opened just a few months before this SARS-CoV-2 virus hit our shores. But our preparations to battle emerging infectious disease outbreaks started way before, after lessons from SARS in 2003. The healthcare system in Singapore put in significant efforts to sustain readiness, with outbreak preparedness drills, expanded laboratory capacity, more isolation rooms, and an emphasis on infection control.

The NCID, as the centre of outbreak response, battled COVID-19 on the frontlines together with Tan Tock Seng Hospital, but this battle soon went beyond our walls, and the entire healthcare system, including acute and community hospitals, private hospitals, and primary care, were activated to fight against COVID-19. Beyond healthcare, a Multi-Ministry Taskforce (MTF) was set up to strategise and coordinate the whole-of-government response to COVID-19, and the MTF is still in operation.

Many months on, we now know more about the virus but it is still evolving. We have strengthened our control strategies, from simple but important public health measures such as mask-wearing, safe distancing measures, and practising good hygiene, to therapeutics and encouraging high rates of vaccination. With good community support, the COVID-19 weekly infection rate in Singapore has stabilised.

The accounts of many involved in the fight against COVID-19 on the clinical, laboratory, epidemiological, research and public health fronts are detailed in this book. I am heartened that they have come together to document this pandemic in Singapore's healthcare history. The virus has impacted the world and no country has been spared. Let us continue to be vigilant and work together to manage COVID-19, not just those of us in the healthcare system but as a nation, and as citizens of the world.

List of Authors by Chapters

1. Professor Leo Yee Sin, Executive Director, National Centre for Infectious Diseases
Adjunct Associate Professor Matthias Paul Toh, Director, National Public Health and Epidemiology Unit, National Centre for Infectious Diseases
Professor David L. Heymann, Professor of Infectious Disease Epidemiology, London School of Hygiene & Tropical Medicine

2. Ms Emma Seow, Manager, Corporate Development, National Centre for Infectious Diseases (till mid-October 2020)
Professor Leo Yee Sin, Executive Director, National Centre for Infectious Diseases

3. Professor Lin-Fa Wang, Professor, Programme in Emerging Infectious Diseases, Duke-NUS Medical School and Faculty, SingHealth Duke-NUS Global Health Institute
Akshamal M. Gamage, PhD, Research Fellow, Programme in Emerging Infectious Diseases, Duke-NUS Medical School
Mr Wharton Chan, MD-PhD Student, Programme in Emerging Infectious Diseases, Duke-NUS Medical School

4. Dr Darius LL Beh, Associate Consultant, National Centre for Infectious Diseases
Professor Dale A Fisher, Senior Consultant, Division of Infectious Diseases, National University Hospital and Professor, Department of Medicine, Yong Loo Lin School of Medicine, National University of Singapore

5. Professor Vernon J Lee, Senior Director, Communicable Diseases Division, Ministry of Health
Dr Calvin J Chiew, Associate Consultant, National Public Health and Epidemiology Unit, National Centre for Infectious Diseases
Dr Zongbin Li, Resident, National University Health System

6. Associate Professor Raymond Lin Tzer Pin, Director, National Public Health Laboratory, National Centre for Infectious Diseases

7. Adjunct Assistant Professor Shawn Vasoo, Clinical Director, National Centre for Infectious Diseases
Adjunct Associate Professor Bernard Thong, Senior Consultant, Department of Rheumatology, Allergy & Immunology and Divisional Chairman (Medicine), Tan Tock Seng Hospital
Dr Margaret Soon, Director of Nursing, National Centre for Infectious Diseases
Adjunct Assistant Professor Ang Hou, Senior Consultant and Head of Emergency Department, Tan Tock Seng Hospital
Mr Albert Tan, Director of Operations, National Centre for Infectious Diseases
Adjunct Associate Professor Tan Hui Ling, Senior Consultant, Department of Anaesthesiology, Intensive Care & Pain Medicine, Assistant Chairman Medical Board (Quality and Clinical Governance), and Chairman, Hospital ICU Committee, Tan Tock Seng Hospital
Dr Benjamin Ho, Senior Consultant, Department of Respiratory & Critical Care Medicine, Tan Tock Seng Hospital and Director, NCID Intensive Care Unit

8. Dr Ramona A. Gutierrez, Manager, Pandemic Preparedness Research Coordinating Office, Infectious Disease Research and Training Office, National Centre for Infectious Diseases

9. Associate Professor Steven PL Ooi, Senior Consultant, Infectious Disease Research and Training Office, National Centre for Infectious Diseases and Associate Professor, Saw Swee Hock School of Public Health, National University of Singapore

10. Ms Christine Gao, Deputy Director, Public Health Operations, National Centre for Infectious Diseases
Adjunct Assistant Professor Wong Chen Seong, Senior Consultant, National Centre for Infectious Diseases

11. Assistant Professor Dr Clive Tan, Group Head and Senior Consultant, Force Health Group, Singapore Armed Forces
Associate Professor Dr Iain Tan, Senior Consultant, Division of Medical Oncology, National Cancer Centre Singapore

Introduction

Professor Leo Yee Sin, Executive Director,
National Centre for Infectious Diseases and
Professor Paul Tambyah, Professor of Medicine,
Infectious Diseases Translational Research Program,
National University of Singapore

The National Centre for Infectious Diseases (NCID) is the result of many years in the planning and finally officially opened its doors in September 2019, just months before the entire world was tested by the COVID-19 pandemic. This book is the work of many people who represent an even larger pool of people from the NCID, Singapore and the rest of the world in trying to understand and contain the SARS-CoV-2 virus at the beginning of the pandemic. There are chapters on science, the public health response, both locally and globally, as well as personal reflections from the NCID and Tan Tock Seng Hospital staff and staff from other public healthcare institutions who were deployed to the NCID, which bring home the human impact of the pandemic. We are very grateful to all the authors for taking the time to put together their thoughtful chapters, as well as the senior academics and public health leaders who have provided us with generous comments on the manuscript. We hope that our readers will gain better insight into the response to the virus from so many different perspectives. Although the pandemic has evolved far beyond the pages of this book globally, the lessons learned from the early days are still relevant. We hope that the chapters will be helpful as we review our experience of this pandemic and face the next emerging infectious disease in the years to come.

1 Overview of the COVID Outbreak in Singapore

Leo Yee Sin, Matthias Paul Toh and David L Heymann

One of the most striking factors of the COVID-19 pandemic has been the variety of response measures taken by countries. Although all implemented mitigation activities such as cancelling large festivals and other events where people gather, some — particularly those in Asia where there were previous SARS or MERS coronavirus outbreaks — applied basic epidemiological principles of outbreak containment that have been known and refined since the mid-19th century. Others applied a mixture of these epidemiological principles and added less precise and more crude principles such as indiscriminately shutting down broad sectors of the economy. Yet others took a different approach and concentrated on motivating their populations to do their own risk assessment and follow government guidance to protect themselves and others.

It is too early to fully evaluate which of these activities have been the most effective in dealing with the COVID-19 pandemic; a more detailed description of country responses can be found in the chapter on global response. Currently, it appears that SARS-CoV-2 is entering an endemic phase, as have four other human coronaviruses that have come before it. Other infectious diseases ranging from tuberculosis to HIV have had the same destiny, and human populations have learnt to live with them.

Although many countries continue to attempt to suppress transmission of the virus to decrease pressure on healthcare systems while waiting for a successful vaccine or therapeutic should they become available, others are taking measures they feel necessary to live with the virus in the long term, as they have learnt from other endemic infections. The response of

Singapore to COVID-19 is a reflection of its preparedness for a pandemic event, having strengthened its level of preparedness and response capacity after the SARS outbreak in 2003.

In addition to having fortified Singapore's National Centre for Infectious Diseases (NCID) with patient care facilities that include state-of-the-art airflow and patient management equipment to ensure effective isolation and care, an intense research programme led to cutting edge technologies in disease detection and alert. It is, therefore, no surprise that early in January 2020, just weeks after the World Health Organization (WHO) reported a cluster of viral pneumonia cases of unknown cause in Wuhan through national focal points of the International Health Regulations, Singapore identified a similar infection in Chinese travellers on 23 January 2020. The immediate response was patient isolation and contact tracing, which successfully contained this initial outbreak. These same measures were applied to other outbreaks that began to occur at various sites in Singapore and became the bedrock to Singapore's epidemiological response to COVID-19 as described in the case study below.

After a long quiet period where infectious diseases of public health significance went under the radar and focus had switched to non-communicable diseases, a novel pathogen known as the Nipah virus crept into Singapore in 1999. This brief outbreak from 11 to 19 March 1999 left behind precious learning points that aided a more organised response in 2003 when the SARS-CoV ravaged many parts of Asia, including Singapore. The 2009 pandemic influenza appeared docile, although many people anticipated another hard hit by an influenza pandemic, as evidenced by constant detection of various zoonotic influenza strains that would threaten the human race. However, many experts were caught off guard by the sudden emergence of another coronavirus with near-perfect human-to-human transmissibility in a short period of time, sparing no continent on earth.

When Wuhan, China, first reported human cases of deadly pneumonia of zoonotic aetiology on 31 December 2019, the world was told to keep calm as there was no evidence of human-to-human transmission. It was hoped that those with direct contact with animals in the implicated marketplace served as dead-end human hosts. However, this belief was proven seriously wrong after family contacts began to fall ill without any exposure to the implicated source. Humans became the perfect vehicles for the virus to move from one place to another within hours.

Situated in the heart of Southeast Asia, Singapore is highly connected to China. Outbreak drawer plans were rehearsed with the clear notion that it would not be spared. However, no one can predict a pandemic's extent or severity. The NCID, which officially opened in September 2019, was tasked with the central role in outbreak response. Being a new purpose-built facility, the NCID has a suite of medical care facilities, complemented with several laboratories that include a National Public Health Laboratory (NPHL), infectious disease research laboratory, and clinical service laboratory. After much anticipation, the first case of COVID-19 was detected in Singapore and reported on 23 January 2020. In Asia, Singapore was the fifth country to detect COVID-19 after Thailand, Japan, South Korea and Vietnam.

The first wave of COVID-19 cases consisted mostly travellers from China, with transmission to local communities, including churches and recreation clubs. The next wave saw the return of young scholars from Europe and the United States after the institutes of higher education that they were studying at either closed or went into lockdown mode. Drastic measures, known as Circuit Breakers (CBs), were implemented to limit human mobility. Around that period, Singapore experienced another mega wave involving migrant workers at dormitories and other types of accommodation housing these workers. By the end of the CB on 1 June 2020, Singapore reported a cumulative total of 52,285 cases by 31 July — 96% of these cases were migrant workers.

Immediate Response

Singapore plunged into setting up a comprehensive range of response actions from public health measures focusing on contact tracing, quarantine and surveillance, to clinical care, including detection, diagnostic, isolation and treatment. On a broader scope, a whole-of-government effort led to the set up of a Multi-Ministry Taskforce anchored by two cabinet ministers (the Ministers for Health and National Development, respectively), with oversight by a Senior Minister, the coordinating minister for emergency response. This section focuses on healthcare responses.

The entire healthcare system was mobilised rapidly. This outbreak witnessed the unity of public health institutions, private providers, primary care providers, and healthcare providers of nursing homes and long-stay facilities. Routine care was severely disrupted and non-urgent treatment was put on hold to focus attention and resources on COVID-19. The NCID plays a pivotal role in several areas: (a) receiving the majority of cases from the community, (b) characterising clinical manifestation, (c) formulating and validating clinical criteria, (d) developing and validating diagnostic tests, (e) providing clinical care including the ICU, and (f) streamlining public health activities with the Communicable Disease Division (CDC) in the Ministry of Health (MOH). Two workgroups — the NCID Therapeutic Workgroup and the national COVID research workgroup — were set up to counter COVID-19, with a simple mission to provide evidence to guide policies on prevention and treatment. Details of their respective work can be found in various chapters of this book.

Key Challenges

It is an understatement on how much disruption, confusion, stress and anxiety a novel pathogen can inflict upon individuals, families, societies and nations. The NCID is a young establishment, and COVID-19 came knocking on its door barely four months after its official opening. In its infancy stage, it appeared to be a mammoth undertaking for the NCID to mount a swift and effective operation. The unity of all sections within the NCID was put to the test.

Confusion and a lack of clear scientific information about the novel disease at the early stage of the epidemic before and soon after the virus reached Singapore compounded the difficulties in mounting effective response actions. The initial early declaration by China that there was no evidence of human-to-human transmission soon gave way to a drastic change in tone when efficient human-to-human transmission by the virus was confirmed. This fuelled suspicion among the international community of the accuracy of the source information and whether there had been any intention to provide misinformation for fear of untoward social circumstances. This further led to disbelief in truthful information, resulting in inappropriate inaction. One such example was the sharing of information about pre-symptomatic transmission. This was generally regarded as an attempt to shift blame on the failure to contain the outbreak.

Perhaps making rational decisions in a time of a crisis shrouded amid uncertainties is part and parcel of dealing with a novel pathogen. Decisions may or may not be borne out simply by relying on past experiences, common knowledge and logic. Therefore, keeping the healthcare system agile and responsive to new findings and knowledge can be frequently overlooked. Risk communication and engagement of all relevant parties including a large majority in the community can be a mammoth task. The wearing of masks among healthy asymptomatic individuals was discouraged at the start of the pandemic. As knowledge accumulated on pre-symptomatic and possibly asymptomatic transmission, the public message flipped to a mandatory wearing of face masks in all public areas. The change in policies based on further knowledge of the characteristics of viral transmission is not wrong. However, the communication has to be succinct, hit the core quickly and bring home the message that wearing a mark prevents transmission and reduces the risk of getting infected. This message has to be internalised by the individual before leading to a self-regulated change in sustainable behaviour, which will take at least a few weeks to adapt to.

Resources were thoroughly stretched as numerous demands arrived from all directions. Indeed, the most precious of all resources was Singapore's healthcare professionals, who valiantly stepped up from the start of the crisis. Hospitals immediately downsized regular care activities, particularly, elective treatments, in order to channel finite resources to combat the outbreak. It was fortunate that the Singapore healthcare system was able to cope with the increased demand to tackle COVID-19. This could have contributed partially to the relatively low mortality rate of COVID-19 deaths in Singapore. The incidence of COVID-19 cases was on a decline at the time of writing. After seven months of putting off regular services, there was a sense of urgency to return service provision to a pre-COVID level. In a way, there was no luxury of time to allow a protracted period of rest. Workforce sustainability remains a priority in outbreak operations.

Along with the COVID-19 epidemic came an "infodemic" that brought an overload of information, of which some lacked credibility. A torrential rush of publications and an unprecedented pre-print and pre-peered review papers flooded the healthcare community. Premature claims of treatment benefits clouded decision-making and the desire to do something may have resulted in more harm than good for the patients. With that in mind, the NCID set up the multi-disciplinary Therapeutic Workgroup that consists of infectious disease physicians, intensivists, immunologists, pharmacists and regulatory specialty to review scientific literature and make suitable conclusions or recommendations for clinical care.

Key Achievements

Singapore's CB imposed significant mobility restrictions that lasted from 7 April to 1 June 2020. At the time of writing, Singapore has entered into Phase 2, post-CB, where a reasonable number of restrictions were relaxed. Workplaces are progressively returning and social gatherings with a small number of participants are allowed. By 31 July, community cases hovered around three per day. The use of facial masks remains mandatory, while social distancing, good hand hygiene, and keeping the environment clean remain key public messages.

Singapore's ability to respond swiftly to the COVID-19 outbreak is a testament to its preparedness during "peace-time", in anticipation of emergencies and readiness to respond when needs arise. Here, we focus the discussion on its healthcare sector.

First, providing adequate isolation facilities to cope with a sudden surge of demand. Singapore's policy to treat all COVID-19 cases until they have made a full recovery and are no longer infectious puts a significant strain on hospital inpatient care facilities. To mitigate this, community care facilities totalling over 18,000 beds were set up in record time at multiple locations across Singapore. Community long-term care facilities and private hospitals were secured by the government. At the height of the epidemic, 19,667 cases were cared for in various isolation facilities.

Second, formulating preventive strategies to enhance surveillance, case detection, contact tracing and testing. The screening of suspect cases first took place at the Screening Centre at the NCID and soon expanded to other public hospitals, polyclinics and community swabbing centres. A diagnosis relied on a real-time polymerase test, where a primer and protocol first developed by the National Public Health Laboratory (NPHL) of the NCID was adopted for use in other hospitals. Fortitude, a locally-developed test kit, was later deployed for testing. A total of 1.4 million PCR-based tests was done at the time of writing, with an aim to reach a testing capacity of 40,000 persons a day. To ensure an adequate supply chain and less reliance on PCR tests, a wide range of products was introduced. There is an impetus for local biotechnology groups to develop tests that can directly detect antigen, thus skipping RNA extraction for PCR. A locally produced serology test, cPass, and other commercially available tests add to Singapore's diagnostic capability.

Third, having the ability to contact trace and quarantine suspect cases to limit transmission. During the post-SARS period, an emphasis on field epidemiological training has progressively enlarged the pool of deployable trained personnel. However, the exponential surge of cases in April 2020 soon overwhelmed the original pool of activity mappers and contact tracers. From early April 2020, the Singapore Armed Forces (SAF) mobilised officers and military experts to be trained in activity mapping and contact tracing. This complemented the resources of the public health institutions and the MOH. Newer tracing technologies and expertise were further enhanced by the expert surveillance investigation team of the Ministry of Home Affairs (MHA). There was a huge demand for the quarantine of close contacts. At the height of the outbreak response, a total of 29,127 people were placed under home quarantine, 592 self-isolated at home while the rest were quarantined in dedicated facilities.

Fourth, emphasising the importance of rapid outbreak research. A Multi-centred Prospective Study To Detect Novel Pathogens And Characterise Emerging Infections (PROTECT) is a pre-formulated protocol approved by the Institutional Review Board (IRB). It had been activated rapidly in response to the outbreak. PROTECT was established at the CDC (the predecessor of the NCID) since 2012. This protocol was put to good use during the Zika outbreak in 2016 and the monkeypox case in 2019. Using a modified form of International Severe Acute Respiratory and Imerging Infection Consortium (ISARIC) (https://isaric.org), PROTECT had been initiated before the arrival of the first case and was in time to establish a longitudinal cohort for 2–3 years of follow-ups. At the time of writing, 571 participants have been recruited into this study. Concurrently the NCID set up the National COVID Research Workgroup with members across all research and academic institutions. The value of this platform was soon recognised and supported by the Chief Health Scientist and National Medical Research Council. Grants were provided to encourage research that could generate evidence to facilitate policy decision-making and have immediate application in disease control and case management. One distinct feature of this collaborative platform is showcasing the unity of the research community against COVID-19.

Fifth, having the ability to apply evidence from research to guide evidence-based clinical care. Several key findings are worth reporting. The quick characterisation of clinical manifestations, including a description of natural disease progression, findings on age-dependent disease severity, and the correlation of viral shedding measured by real-time PCR on upper respiratory samples in relation to disease progression and inference on transmissibility. We soon reckoned that a high viral shedding is detected at the onset of the illness and that this level declines progressively. Pneumonia typically develops during the second week of illness and some patients may require supplementary oxygen, mechanical ventilation or extracorporeal membrane oxygenation (ECMO). Clinical symptoms are generally mild and innocuous at the onset and could progressively become more pronounced. These findings prompted the local policy of having five days of medical leave for self-monitoring and to minimise transmission. The majority of these cases, particularly those below 45 years of age, had uneventful illnesses. In the subsequent large outbreak involving young foreign workers, age was effectively used to triage the level of care. The majority of them were cared for in community care facilities. Of the 27 death cases reported by end-July, the median age was 73 years (range: 41–97).

Sixth, a low incidence rate among healthcare workers. There is emerging local evidence suggesting that these workers have a lower incidence rate than other occupational groups. Several possible reasons could explain this: Good infection control practices, adequate personal protective equipment (PPE) supply, a safe working environment, better knowledge and skills to protect themselves, etc.

The COVID-19 case mortality rate in Singapore remains among the lowest globally, at about 5 per 100,000 persons in a population. Multiple factors could have contributed to that: the early detection and admission of all PCR-confirmed cases allowed for close monitoring and early intervention, the setting up of a therapeutic workgroup to appraise the rapidly evolving therapeutic landscape and the convalescent plasma program, putting patients in a prone position (serious cases were admitted to the ICU when signs of respiratory strain appeared), an adequate ICU capacity, planned elective intubation to prevent crash landing, access to an antiviral agent such as remdesivir in international trials, etc., are all factors that could have contributed to the favourable outcome in different degrees. The ICU mortality rate in Singapore has been hovering around 14%.

Building Community Resilience

COVID-19 presents itself as an unprecedented challenge to humankind. The elusive nature of the virus leaves behind many unresolved questions; its impact is not only felt by the healthcare sector but jocks the entire social fabric and has done tremendous damage to the global economy. It accentuates and exposes inequality, sparing no individual or society, and nations have to re-shape and adjust to new ways of living. The Singapore government made a conscious, calculated move to mobilise about S$100 billion to tide the nation through the COVID-19 pandemic, of which S$52 billion was drawn from past national reserves. The S$6.4-billion support in the Unity Budget was followed by the Resilience (S$48.4 billion), Solidarity (S$5.1 billion) and Fortitude (S$33 billion) budgets. A fifth support package (S$8 billion) was announced at the August Ministerial Statement. Beyond funding Singapore's public health response, these five COVID support packages also provide stimuli to resuscitate the badly affected economic sectors and create and sustain job opportunities.

Moving Forward

Globalisation has accelerated the spread of the SARS-CoV-2 virus that has spared no country in the seven months since its discovery. The exponential increase of cases in all continents has been partially controlled after the shutting down of borders, mandating the use of masks, maintaining safe social distance and restricting human movement. However, new cases are expected to return upon the easing of these non-sustainable measures. Although a vaccine has been widely expected to be the only definitive solution to this COVID-19 pandemic, it remains uncertain when this vaccine will be available and accessible to the masses. There is also no promise that such a vaccine will be safe and effective in protecting the vulnerable whose altered immunity system inherently weakens the body's ability to mount a response to the vaccine. Adverse effects and the durability of the vaccine also remain untested. Recent reports of remdesivir, an antivirus, and a low dose of dexamethasone have shown a beneficial effect in severe cases who needed supplementary oxygen or mechanical ventilation. The overall paucity of consistent data still requires further research to examine the reproducibility and transmissibility of the SARS-CoV-2 virus. In the interim, while waiting for an effective vaccine and therapeutic approach, we can only rely on non-pharmaceutical preventive measures to limit the spread of SARS-CoV-2.

References

Bagdasarian N, Fisher D. (2020) Heterogeneous COVID-19 transmission dynamics within Singapore: A clearer picture of future national responses. *BMC Medicine* **18**:164. https://doi.org/10.1186/s12916-020-01625-7

Crosby JC, Heimann MA, Burleson SL *et al.* (2020) COVID-19: A review of therapeutics under investigation. JACEP Open 1–7. https://doi.org/10.1002/emp2.12081

Dickens BL, Koo JR, Wilder-Smith A *et al.* (2020) Institutional, not hone-based, isolation could contain the COVID-19 outbreak. *Lancet* 1541–42.

Lurie N *et al.* (2020) Developing COVID-19 vaccine at pandemic speed. *N Eng J Med* **382**:1969–73.

Ng YX, Li ZB, Chua YX *et al.* (2020) Evaluation of the effectiveness of surveillance and containment measures of the first 100 patients with COVID-19 in Singapore — January 2–February 29. *Morb Mortal W Rep* **69**(11):307–11.

Paton NI, Leo YS, Zaki SR *et al.* (1999) Outbreak of Nipah virus infection among abattoir workers in Singapore. *Lancet* **354**:1253–56.

Pung R, Chiew CJ, Young BE *et al.* (2020) Investigation of three clusters of COVID-19 in Singapre: Implications for surveillance and response measures. *Lancet* **395**:1039–46.

Wei WE, Li ZB, Chiew CJ *et al.* (2020) Presymptomatic transmission of SARS-CoV-2 — Singapore, January 23–March 16. *Morb Mortal W Rep* **69**(14):411–15.

Wong JEL, Leo YS, Tan CC. (2020) COVID-19 in Singapore — Current experience. Critical global issues that require attention and action. *JAMA* **323**(13): 1243–44. doi:10.1001/jama.2020.2467

Young BE, Ong EW, Kalimuddin S *et al.* (2020) Epidemiologic features and clinical course of patients infected with SARS-CoV-2 in Singapore. *JAMA* **323**(15): 1488–94. doi:10.100/jama.2020.3204

Zagury-Orly I *et al.* (2020) COVID-19 — a reminder to reason. *N Eng J Med* **383**:e12.

2 Introducing the NCID

Emma Seow and Leo Yee Sin

Why Singapore Needs a New Dedicated Infectious Disease Facility

As a densely populated and strategically located trade and travel hub with porous borders, Singapore is unique and, as a result, faces a number of distinctive challenges. It is home to 5.7 million people, of which 28% (or 1.6 million) are non-citizens or permanent residents, and caters to an annual tourist volume of approximately three times the size of its population. While its popularity as a business and leisure travel destination has greatly encouraged trade and economic growth, this also makes the small city-state highly susceptible to emerging infectious diseases from other parts of the world. In addition, Singapore's high population density of more than 8,000 people per square metre means that once individuals contract certain droplet or airborne infections, these can spread quickly to a large number of people if cases are not swiftly isolated or contained.

With globalisation, we have to face the reality that emerging infections are the norm today. As seen from a series of global epidemics ranging from MERS-CoV to H1N1 and even the recent imported case of monkeypox, emerging pathogen epidemics are a major public health concern. The Communicable Disease Centre (CDC) at Moulmein Road once catered to the treatment of patients with infectious diseases, weathering early outbreaks and having its facilities repurposed for more recent challenges such as Nipah, SARS and Zika. Singapore's healthcare infrastructure has evolved since the CDC was built in 1913, and so too have the demands made on our healthcare institutions and the threats of infectious diseases. It is thus timely for the century-old well-served facility to land a new home furnished with the latest technologies.

Planning for an Infectious Disease Centre to Serve the Needs of Our Population

When SARS hit Singapore in 2003, significant healthcare resources had to be channelled towards fighting the outbreak, including the closure of one of Singapore's busiest hospitals, Tan Tock Seng Hospital (TTSH), which became the designated screening and treatment centre for SARS. This meant that the healthcare system on the whole had less capacity to cater to routine healthcare needs, particularly non-communicable chronic medical illnesses. The take-home lesson? It was thus important for Singapore to have a dedicated centre with the capacity to accommodate a medium-size outbreak such as SARS, and to be flexible enough to scale-up capacity should the number of suspect and confirmed cases escalate.

In addition, an important factor to consider is to have a self-contained full suite of services on-site. This concept is to enable a lockdown of the facility during a major outbreak or pandemic and yet be self-sufficient to provide optimal care with no or minimal movement of cases.

Simultaneously, while the new infectious disease centre needs to be fully-equipped to handle infectious disease outbreaks and pandemics, it is equally important for the centre to provide routine infectious disease treatment and "peace-time" public health functions.

Design Principles

Knowledge gained from lessons experienced during the 2003 SARS outbreak and other outbreaks were integral to the development and design of the state-of-the-art facility that now sits in the centre of the HealthCity Novena Campus. The 14-storey National Centre for Infectious Diseases (NCID) building is built on five design principles — Safety, Capacity and Scalability, Capability, Convertibility and Connectivity.

Safety

The safety of the NCID's patients, staff and that of the general public are of utmost priority. To achieve this, the NCID building is designed to ensure there is a clear segregation of airflow, waste, materials and people movement.

The 14-storey building is divided into two: a low-risk wing on the left and a high-risk wing on the right. Each floor contains separate pathways and dedicated lifts for patients, visitors and staff, and facilitates the flow of clean and dirty material movement to prevent the mixing and contamination across groups.

A key feature of the centre pays special attention to airflow and circulation in and out of the building. Through a single pass air conditioning system, there is a separate air handling unit (AHU) for each ward, supplying clean air to the different zones on each floor: the low-risk area, the high-risk area and the visitor area. The exhaust system is fitted with a top-tiered High Efficiency Particulate Air (HEPA) filter, through which air from patients' room will pass through before being released as clean air into the surrounding environment.

Likewise, waste management processes at the NCID comply with international and local regulations and standards. Patient waste is thoroughly decontaminated before being discharged to the public sewer.

Capacity and scalability

The NCID is a 17-ward hospital built to contain 330 beds — the number of beds required during SARS, which was considered a medium-size outbreak, with the option for capacity ramp-up and scalability for larger pandemics. The rooms in the NCID include 64 cohort beds, 100 isolation rooms, 124 negative pressure rooms, 38 intensive care unit (ICU) beds and 4 High-Level Isolation Unit (HLIU) beds. This allows the NCID to cater to the population of Singapore during "peace-time" and outbreaks, as well as a wide range of endemic and imported infectious diseases.

Capability

The NCID building has a full spectrum of clinical care facilities within the NCID building, so as to provide patients with a full range of care on-site while minimising patient movement, especially for those with highly infectious conditions. In addition, having these services — inpatient facilities, diagnostic radiology, operating theatres, an outpatient clinic, laboratories and a screening centre — within the building would improve the NCID's functionality should a lockdown occur.

The NCID is home to the first and only purpose-built special HLIU in Singapore with enhanced facilities for managing patients with suspected or confirmed infections involving High-Level Isolation Pathogens such as Ebola or other viral hemorrhagic fevers. The unit has been carefully designed in terms of space, material and person flow, airflow and waste management to ensure the safety of all users of the unit and the building. It is also equipped with macerators and hydrogen peroxide vaporisers for specialised decontamination and waste management. Key features of the HLIU include an on-site laboratory, which allows for the prompt processing of patient samples, and autoclave facilities. Each room is further equipped with ventilators and dialysis capabilities. The HLIU is staffed by a highly trained core team of infectious disease and ICU doctors, nurses and healthcare workers dedicated to providing patient care that requires special attention to biosafety; staff working in the HLIU are specially trained to don and carry out clinical work in their Personal Protective Equipment (PPE), which includes a water impermeable gown and Powered Air-Purifying Respirator (PAPR).

In addition, the NCID has a 4,980 square metre purpose-built Screening Centre (SC) that can be activated during outbreaks for mass screening. The SC has dedicated drop-off access and is segregated into low and high-risk zones. The capabilities of the SC are supplemented by the outpatient clinic with a Special Precaution Area (SPA), which has the capability to handle a small outbreak. During "peace-time", patients visiting the clinic and identified as requiring isolation precautions will be escorted to the

SPA, where all services will be rendered within the area by staff wearing PPE, to minimise patient movement.

Convertibility

The NCID is built for greater functional flexibility, which will allow its facilities to be used for various purposes during "peace-time". To retain surge capacity, approximately one-third of the wards are kept empty. These spaces are utilised for training, innovative research and other purposes.

Another example is the NCID SC that is built with minimal fixed structures, which enables the space to be used for a wide range of activities, including workshops, training and even events such as the NCID official opening and year-end party for the staff.

The HLIU has been used as a space for training and drills regularly during "peace-time" to accustom staff to carrying out their clinical work in the exact space and conditions that they will be working in should the HLIU be activated.

Connectivity

In order to facilitate the efficient and effective provision of care and services to patients, the NCID is located at the centre of the HealthCity Novena Campus and is well-connected to TTSH via a series of sky bridges as well as a pedestrian concourse, underpass, Automated Guide Vehicle (AGV) service tunnel and vehicle link. This allows the easy transfer of patients with infectious conditions from TTSH Emergency Department to the NCID, the movement of healthcare workers from other specialties, and the transportation of equipment and shared services to the NCID.

The NCID is connected via sky bridges to the Ng Teng Fong Centre for Healthcare Innovation and the Lee Kong Chian School of Medicine (LKC Medicine), thus facilitating collaboration between NCID healthcare workers and the professors, deans, researchers and academics at LKC Medicine. This invigorating sharing of ideas will lead to more breakthroughs in infectious disease research and capability development in academic training and education.

The Organisational Structure of the NCID: An Example of Integration of Clinical Management with Public Health Units, Academic Research and Training

Clinical diagnosis, treatment and management are key to Singapore's integrated response to emerging infections and outbreaks, but they need to be coupled with **public health surveillance systems** and **academic research and training** for a revised and expanded framework to fortify Singapore's readiness efforts against the substantial global infectious disease threats of today.

The NCID's core public health units include the National Public Health and Epidemiology Unit (NPHEU), the National Public Health Laboratory (NPHL) and the Antimicrobial Resistance Coordinating Office. Further to that, the NCID plays a role in driving major public health goals such as those identified by disease-specific national health initiatives for HIV/AIDs and tuberculosis through coordinating the National Public Health programmes for HIV and tuberculosis.

One of the most important factors to staying vigilant against the threat of infectious diseases is the provision of relevant and scientifically valid epidemiologic data to base decisions and policies on. The NPHEU actively supports the Ministry of Health (MOH) by providing recommendations for national strategies for the prevention and control of communicable diseases. The team is responsible for long-term horizon scanning and risk assessment of infectious disease threats for clinical and public health practice guidance.

Another key entity within the NCID is a system of diagnostic and reference laboratories actively involved in the laboratory surveillance and preparedness for highly infectious pathogens, such as MERS-CoV, H7N9 and Ebola. The NPHL is essential for conducting laboratory-based surveillance of infectious diseases and provides specialised diagnostic tests that track changes in existing organisms, detect novel and re-emerging pathogens and respond to outbreaks. The NPHL has been involved in past outbreak investigations, including the Chikungunya outbreak in 2008, the H1N1 pandemic in 2009 and the Zika outbreak in 2016. The streamlined workflow within the NCID has successfully established the efficient and safe transfer of infectious biologic samples from a clinical ward to the NPHL within 30 minutes. A recent monkeypox case attests to the record speed that was demonstrated from receiving the case to an isolation room, clinical assessments, sample collection for testing and reaching a definitive diagnosis using multiple primer sets of PCR, electron microscopy of the first case of monkeypox in Asia within 30 hours

Facilities at the NPHL include a biosafety-level 3 containment facility that is dedicated to the surveillance of infections of public health importance as well as the detection and identification of novel pathogens. The NPHL uses the best science for the laboratory surveillance of infectious diseases and the investigation of outbreaks, and is one of the network of specialised Electron Microscopy laboratories in the world trained and prepared to look at Risk Group 3 and Emerging Infectious Disease (EID) agents.

Singapore's response to the infectious disease threats of today cannot depend solely on clinical and public health management. Academic inquiry is part of the bigger plan of how we strive to be a national leader in infectious disease management. To guard against Singapore's vulnerability amidst rising challenges, our public health and scientific community work hand-in-hand to co-lead our research capabilities in gathering new knowledge on novel pathogens, and to increase the translational impact of our research. The pursuit of more evidence-based clinical management and therapies will enable effective mitigation strategies in both containment and treatment of infectious diseases in our community.

The National Infectious Disease Research Coordinating Office (NIDRCO) and NCID Research Office, both under the Infectious Disease Research and Training Office (IDRTO), oversee research and research facilities at the NCID. The IDRCO reviews the strategy and general direction for ID research in Singapore, including Pandemic Preparedness Research, and encourages collaborative clinical infectious disease research and outbreak research between healthcare institutions in Singapore and the region. Assisting the nation in building a strong response infrastructure, the team also develops human capital for ID research through seed funding and travel fellowships. The NCID Research Office conducts a wide range of infectious disease research in emerging infectious diseases and routine conditions such as dengue and other vector-borne diseases, antimicrobial resistance, tropical medicine, HIV and nosocomial infections with the use of NCID's in-house research clinic and research laboratory.

Our healthcare workers are the key to disease outbreak readiness and will thus have to stay up to date with the latest skills and competencies to ensure the highest level of expertise. Under the Training and Education Office of the IDRTO, the NCID extensively trains and develops the capabilities of healthcare workers. Since 2018, the NCID has been progressively carrying out disease outbreak readiness training consisting of drills and exercises. These include campus-wide and inter-cluster collaborations to build professional capabilities in regional health systems and Intermediate and Long-Term Care (ILTC) providers.

Looking Back and Looking Ahead: Moving from the CDC to NCID, NCID Official Opening and Today

Set up by the MOH, the NCID is Singapore's dedicated national-level entity that serves as the leading authority in infectious disease management, coupled with an in-house public health unit to fulfil the national mandates in the fight against infectious diseases. Tapping on the clinical governance of TTSH, it allows a full range of integrated clinical services from other specialities.

The services at the new NCID facility began operating in phases starting from November 2018 with all services fully functioning by May 2019. Shortly after its move, the team at the NCID had to face the challenge of treating the first imported case of monkeypox in May 2019, which was successfully contained, diagnosed and treated without secondary transmission. The HLIU was once activated involving a case of severe malaria with initial suspicion of Ebola. The NCID team had a chance to put their skills to the test and carry out their national mission.

The NCID officially opened on 7 September 2019. Barely four months later, COVID-19 arrived in Singapore. The NCID is further challenged by this unprecedented nature of outbreak to play a leading role in the country's efforts to contain and treat the disease, which are detailed in the subsequent chapters of this book.

3 Role of Animals in the COVID-19 Outbreak

Lin-Fa Wang[1,2], Akshamal M Gamage[1] and Wharton Chan[1]

Introduction

The novel coronavirus SARS-CoV-2 is the causative agent of COVID-19, a pneumonia-like disease which first emerged in Wuhan, China, in late 2019, and spread rapidly around the world. The disease has a broad range of severity, ranging from asymptomatic infections, mild flu-like symptoms to acute-respiratory distress syndrome and death (Guan *et al.*, 2020; Huang *et al.*, 2020; Young *et al.*, 2020).

Zoonoses are defined as infections that have a non-human animal source, and occur at the interface between humans and animals, such as during livestock farming, trading of exotic animals and bush-meat consumption. The majority of novel human pathogens in the last century have been documented to be zoonotic in origin (Jones *et al.*, 2008; Taylor *et al.*, 2001). Zoonotic diseases often involve an animal reservoir species that is capable of hosting the virus asymptomatically. Most, if not all, human coronaviruses identified prior to SARS-CoV-2 are of animal origin, including the SARS-CoV outbreak in 2003 from bats to humans via civet cats (Guan *et al.*, 2003), and the MERS-CoV outbreak in 2012, which is transmitted to humans from dromedary camels (Alagaili *et al.*, 2014), and is also thought to have originated in bats (Cui *et al.*, 2019). Other bat-borne viruses include

[1] Programme in Emerging Infectious Diseases, Duke-NUS Medical School, Singapore
[2] SingHealth Duke-NUS Global Health Institute, Singapore
Correspondence email: linfa.wang@duke-nus.edu.sg

Nipah, Hendra and rabies viruses (Calisher *et al.*, 2006). Various other animals have also been linked to important diseases of zoonotic origin, such as waterfowl, as reservoirs for Influenza A viruses (Taubenberger & Kash, 2010) and primates for HIV (Sharp & Hahn, 2011).

Most zoonotic infections are not capable of efficient human-to-human transmission, and therefore cause limited infections in the human population (Parrish *et al.*, 2008). Various barriers can limit the efficiency of human-to-human transmission after zoonotic spillover, such as poor entry-receptor compatibility, varied entry-receptor tissue distribution patterns, and the inability to withstand or antagonise human immune-responses. In the event the pathogen is able to acquire mutations for human-adaptation and transmission, the absence of prior immunity leads to the rapid spread of the virus among the human population. The encroachment of human activity into wildlife habitats, global interconnectedness, and increasing human density have all contributed to an increased frequency of pathogen emergence, and with it, an increased risk of human adaptation and subsequent spread by viruses of zoonotic origin.

While identifying the causative agent for a zoonotic disease is the first step of an outbreak investigation and is greatly facilitated by modern discovery tools such as next generation sequencing (NGS), confident attribution to the zoonotic mode of spillover is significantly more complicated. This is partly because of uncertain links between a reservoir host, and one or more intermediate species, before transmission happens to humans. The exact occurrence of the initial transmission event is often difficult to pinpoint, as public health attention is usually drawn to clusters or spikes in cases, which can manifest after a significant period of undetected human-human transmission. If intermediate host species are involved in the transmission of the virus from the reservoir host to humans, there could be sporadic batches of animals infected upon contact with the reservoir host, and extensive screening would be required to identify successful matches. When the virus species is capable of genetic recombination, as is common in the case of coronaviruses (Su *et al.*, 2016), multiple animal species may have related virus strains with different genome segments having homology to the zoonotic virus of interest, giving rise to complex mosaic ancestries. On top of such, data acquisition and analyses require OneHealth teams of cross-disciplinary scientists at the suspected region of spillover, which can be complicated by geopolitical, economic, institutional and cultural factors.

Bats and SARS-CoV-2

Several zoonoses have been linked to *Chiroptera* (bats) as the reservoir host (Wang & Anderson, 2019). Bats are a highly abundant and diverse group of mammals, making up roughly 20% of all known mammalian species (Teeling *et al.*, 2018). The reasons underlining the significantly higher viral diversity in bats are not yet fully understood, but have been attributed to the species richness of this mammalian order (Olival *et al.*, 2017), as well as to an altered immune response (Brook & Dobson, 2015; O'Shea *et al.*, 2014; Pavlovich *et al.*, 2018; Zhang *et al.*, 2013). The latter is linked to another attribute in bats unique amongst mammals — powered flight. The evolution of powered flight is hypothesised to have necessitated an increased tolerance of the bat immune system to physiological stressors and endogenous damage associated molecular patterns (DAMPs), which would have incidental effects on the host response during viral infections (Ahn *et al.*, 2019).

Coronaviruses can be phylogenetically classified into four genera, and coronavirus species linked to human infections have to date been identified only from the genera *Alphacoronavirus* and *Betacoronavirus* (Cui *et al.*, 2019). Bats have been observed to host a remarkable diversity of alpha and beta-coronaviruses (Wong *et al.*, 2019; Woo *et al.*, 2012). SARS-related coronaviruses (SARSr-CoVs) have been detected most frequently in bats of the genus *Rhinolophus*, particularly from Chinese horseshoe bats (*Rhinolophus sinicus*) (Hu *et al.*, 2017; Lau *et al.*, 2005). Longitudinal sampling of bats in a cave in Yunnan, China, over a period of ten years identified multiple SARSr-CoVs that have various gene segments highly similar to that of SARS-CoV (Hu *et al.*, 2017). Recombination events within the co-circulating pool of CoVs in this cave are postulated to have given rise to the direct precursor of SARS-CoV (Hu *et al.*, 2017). SARSr-CoVs were identified in this location, which have spike protein sequences with near-identical receptor-binding domains (RBD) to the original SARS-CoV, and which utilise the same host-receptor, angiotensin converting enzyme 2 (ACE2) (Ge *et al.*, 2013).

Importantly, the closest identified relative to date for SARS-CoV-2, RaTG13 (Fig. 1), was detected from a *Rhinolophus* bat and shared a 96% genomic sequence identity to SARS-CoV-2, pointing to a potential bat origin for this coronavirus species as well (Zhou *et al.*, 2020b). Spike proteins from both SARS-CoV-2 and RaTG13 spike proteins are capable of binding the ACE2 receptor (Shang *et al.*, 2020; Zhou *et al.*, 2020b). An important difference between these two proteins is that the RaTG13 spike

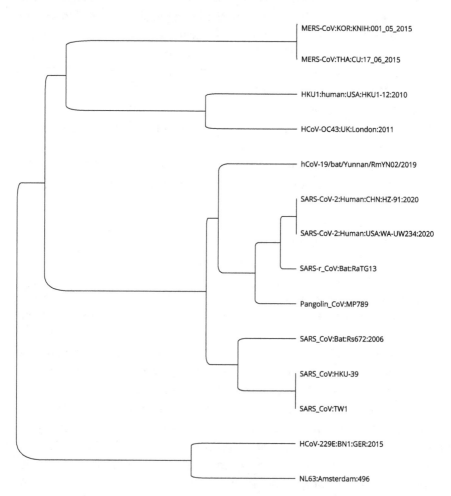

Figure 1.   Phylogenetic tree of the spike gene sequence from various alpha- and beta-coronaviruses. Sequences acquired from GenBank and GISAID, aligned with MAFFT (Nakamura *et al.*, 2018), followed by tree building using BEAST v1.10.4 (Suchard *et al.*, 2018), with HKY substitution model (Hasegawa *et al.*, 1985) and an Expansion Growth Tree Prior (Griffiths & Tavare, 1994), 10000000 MCMC Chain Length and 1000000 burn-in.

protein lacks a polybasic cleavage site between the S1/S2 domains on the spike protein, the presence of which has been reported to contribute to the infectivity of SARS-CoV-2, via enabling spike protein processing by ubiquitous host furin proteases (Andersen *et al.*, 2020; Coutard *et al.*, 2020; Hoffmann *et al.*, 2020; Shang *et al.*, 2020; Walls *et al.*, 2020). Although polybasic cleavage sites have been detected in species from both alpha- and betacoronaviruses previously (Millet & Whittaker, 2015), SARS-CoV-2 represents the first member of the "lineage B" clade of betacoronaviruses to possess this amino acid sequence (Andersen *et al.*, 2020; Coutard *et al.*, 2020). A recent report subsequently identified a bat CoV closely related to SARS-CoV-2, RmYN02 (Fig. 1), isolated from *Rhinolophus malayensis*, which had three amino acid insertions at the S1/S2 junction (Zhou *et al.*, 2020a). It remains to be seen whether future sampling work uncovers lineage B betacoronaviruses with polybasic insertion sites circulating in *Rhinolophus* bats. For SARS-CoV, it took almost ten years to find its ancestor virus in bats (Ge *et al.*, 2013). Extensive and long-term virus surveillance efforts in suspected animal reservoirs are likely to be required in order to fully reconstruct the recombination events that gave rise to a more recent precursor of SARS-CoV-2 in bats.

Is There an Intermediate Animal Host(s) Involved in the COVID-19 Outbreak?

Intermediate hosts can act as conduits between the reservoir host and the human population. Live-animal markets where wildlife and livestock are sold have received increased attention recently. The close proximity between animals and humans in these markets, and the natural generation of biological fluids from animals during the culling and trading process can significantly increase the risk of zoonotic transmission from infected animals that were previously exposed to the reservoir host. The live-animal markets in Southern China were also previously linked to the origin of the SARS-CoV outbreak (Guan *et al.*, 2003). Early during the COVID-19 pandemic, the Huanan Seafood Market in Wuhan, China, was identified as a potential site of concern (Normile, 2020). However, analysis of data from the first 41 patients in China revealed that although the majority (66%) of patients had exposure to the market place, 13 patients had no links to that place

(Huang *et al.*, 2020). It is therefore unclear if the market was the site of a spillover event or of an early super-spreading event from human patients who had contacted the disease elsewhere. In the absence of an exact site of spillover being identified, the list of potential intermediate hosts becomes very broad. However, as intermediate hosts often have close contact with humans, understanding if any such species were involved in SARS-CoV-2 zoonosis is of significant importance to prevent recurrent spillover events. One approach could entail the use of sequence conservation analysis for entry-associated host proteins in various animal species (Damas *et al.*, 2020; Liu *et al.*, 2020; Wong *et al.*, 2020), together with an evaluation of their geographical distribution, ecological niches and potential interactions with humans, in order to provide a framework for identifying animal species that have the potential to be intermediate hosts during the SARS-CoV-2 outbreak. This could then be followed by more extensive surveillance within this narrowed list of animals, including viral metagenomics sequencing and serological analysis.

Thus far, Malayan pangolins (*Manis javanica*) are the only non-bat species in which CoVs closely related to SARS-CoV-2 have been identified (Lam *et al.*, 2020; Xiao *et al.*, 2020). Of interest, the spike protein RBD on pangolin CoVs were nearly identical to that of SARS-CoV-2 (97.4% amino acid identity), and had a higher amino acid sequence identity than bat CoV RaTG13 RBD (Lam *et al.*, 2020). However, the rest of the pangolin CoV genome regions showed a greater degree of divergence from SARS-CoV-2 compared to RaTG13 (Lam *et al.*, 2020; Xiao *et al.*, 2020). While these findings raise the possibility of SARS-CoV-2 RBD acquisition from pangolin CoVs via recombination, they do not convincingly support the role of pangolins as an intermediate species carrying a direct precursor to SARS-CoV-2. Rather, they highlight the as-of-yet under-sampled diversity of coronaviruses in mammalian hosts and indicate the possibility that other mammalian species too can act as hosts to SARS-CoV-2 or related viruses.

Transmission and Molecular Epidemiology

The ability to acquire virus sequences in short time frames and with relative ease has vastly changed the response to this pandemic, as compared to SARS-CoV in 2003. From the first sequence published in early January 2020 from Wuhan, China (Zhu *et al.*, 2020), to the date of writing (20 June 2020), close to 3,000 genomes have been deposited in the GISAID database (https://www.gisaid.org/). This resource has been invaluable in conducting phylogenetic studies, and indirectly providing information to public health authorities to make informed decisions (Eden *et al.*, 2020).

Early in the outbreak, many regional sequences were published along with phylogenetic studies in order to understand the primary question of *"where the virus came from"* (Castillo *et al.*, 2020; Eden *et al.*, 2020; Lu *et al.*, 2020a; Zehender *et al.*, 2020). In these types of studies, the primary goal was to cross reference genetic data and travel histories to track transmission chains. The conclusions in this type of study, especially early in the outbreak, however, may sometimes be limiting due to the lack of data available. For example, in a study where three sequences were reported (Zehender *et al.*, 2020), from Italy, the authors were unable to trace beyond the closest source in Europe by phylogenetics, and backed their conclusion with other epidemiological data.

As the number of sequenced genomes increases, phylogenetic network type analysis become more informative in looking at a more global picture and working out more complex transmission chains (Forster *et al.*, 2020; Yu *et al.*, 2020). The advantage of these analyses is that it allows extra depth in reconstructing transmission chains, and also uses agnostically derived nodes to inform relationships between sequences that otherwise cannot be shown in classic trees. Additionally, these networks provide extra insights on classic epidemiology questions such as the geographical source of the virus. As discussed above, the original notion that the virus started its spread from the Wuhan Huanan Seafood Market has since been challenged due to the questionable epidemiological links (Huang *et al.*, 2020), with 13 of the 41 reported cases having no links to the market. Indeed, using haplotype-based phylogenetic networks, sequences linked to the market were shown to be derived from substitution of another widely circulating haplotype in Wuhan, which therefore concludes that the virus did not *originate* from the market (Yu *et al.*, 2020). Interestingly, the market-linked haplotype was shown to be more widespread than the claimed ancestral haplotype, though the authors did suggest the possibility of under-sampling of early cases that were not linked to the market.

Genomic Diversity and Evolution

Another key question that phylogenetic studies allow us to look into is the diversity of the different viral sequences over the course of time, thus the mutation rate. The mutation rate, however, is difficult to experimentally determine, so is often proxied by evolutionary rates (for the short term) and substitution rates (for the long term) (Holmes *et al.*, 2016). Looking at substitution rates, SARS-CoV-2 is shown to have $0.14 - 1.31 \times 10^{-3}$ substitutions per site per year (Rambaut, 2020) compared to $0.14 - 1.1 \times 10^{-3}$ in MERS (Cotten *et al.*, 2013) and $0.80 - 2.38 \times 10^{-3}$ in SARS-CoV (Zhao *et al.*, 2004), which is comparable or lower than the other two coronaviruses. When compared to other RNA viruses, this rate is even more unremarkable (Holmes *et al.*, 2016), and this may be explained by the presence of a proofreading exonuclease nsp14 in SARS-CoV-2. However, due to the nature of it being an RNA virus, the lower levels of mutation rates will to some extent be compensated by high replication rates, and substitution rates are projected to fall within the distribution of RNA viruses (Zhang & Holmes, 2020).

Looking at overall viral genomic diversity in a geographical fashion may also provide insight as to whether the virus has increased mutations, possibly due to different selective pressures in different regions. In a phylogenetic network analysis, mutations were only found outside of East Asia for a particular cluster derived in the network (Forster *et al.*, 2020), but the authors also noted a problem in this type of analysis: most of the Chinese sequences were sequenced during the early part of the outbreak. The time, and the number of samples sequenced, can hugely impact signals from different geographical regions. Indeed, some have noted that the genomic diversity is roughly the same across the globe, with the exception of China and to an extent, Italy, and this could be due to under-sampling together with an early temporal element.

Diversity can also be looked in a more micro perspective, interrogating the rates at which individual genes, and even nucleotides, are more prone to substitution, and the functional consequences of such. There are three kinds of nucleotide changes that are in play here: purifying/negative selection, positive selection and recombination. The strength of these pressures all depend on the region; for example, nsp1 and nsp3 have been shown to have the weakest constraints, with ORF8 shown to be at selection neutrality (Cagliani *et al.*, 2020). Particular attention has been placed on the S1 protein, which contains the receptor binding motif. Positive selection analysis has shown this to be a hotspot (Cagliani *et al.*, 2020), and S1 has also shown to be a strong homoplasic site (independent parallel mutation prone) (van Dorp *et al.*, 2020). However, caution must be exercised in this region due to a possibility of a recombination event, even though both articles showed no evidence of recombination. In order to detect a recombination event, more sequences from the primary host and hypothetical intermediate host are required (Zhang & Holmes, 2020), and thus remains to be seen.

There has been considerable debate in the functional correlation of particular strains, as to whether adapted/mutated strains will cause a change in phenotype, such as increased transmissibility and virulence. Early in the outbreak, Tang *et al.* (2020b) described the S and L type theory and claimed that there are different transmission rates between the two. This has been fiercely rebutted by others with no consensus as of yet. More recently, the D614G mutation in the Spike protein has attracted great attention. Although the mutation is located outside the RBD, the virus variant has shown increasing representation in the published genomes and the mutation has been postulated to potentially confer structural advantage to the furin cleavage domain (Tang *et al.*, 2020a) and increase viral infectivity (Hu *et al.*, 2020). It is premature to make claims on a change in phenotype based on phylogenetic, structural or epidemiologic data alone without experimental validation. As for other phenotypic characteristics, such as virulence, some believe that the virus would more likely adapt to be more transmissible, but would unlikely precipitate in more virulence (Grubaugh *et al.*, 2020).

Spillback or Reverse Zoonotic Potential

The ability of the SARS-CoV-2 spike protein to bind ACE2 receptors from a broad range of mammalian species (Liu *et al.*, 2020) (Table 1), coupled with the rapid spread of SAR-CoV-2 in the human population, has raised the possibility of reverse zoonosis among animal populations in contact

Table 1. Amino acid sequence identity of key receptor and accessory host proteins for SARS-CoV-2 entry (%)

	ACE2	TMPRSS2	FURIN	NRP1
Homo sapiens	100*	100	100	100
Mus musculus	82#	78	94	93
Macaca mulatta	95*	88	99	99
Rousettus aegypticus	79*	77	94	94
Rhinolophus ferrumequinum	80*	81	91	95
Sus scrofa	81*	77	94	96
Manis javanica	85*	78	90	95
Mustela putorius furo	83*	73	96	96

Symbols denote that orthologous ACE2 expression can (*) or cannot (#) mediate viral entry upon over-expression in cells (*Liu et al.* PNAS 2021, https://doi.org/10.1073/pnas.2025373118).

with humans (Gryseels *et al.*, 2020). As shown in Table 2, experimental *in-vivo* infection studies have demonstrated a growing range of species, including hamsters, primates, ferrets, fruit bats, cats and dogs as being permissive for infection with SARS-CoV-2 (Chan *et al.*, 2020; Lu *et al.*, 2020b; Munster *et al.*, 2020; Schlottau *et al.*, 2020; Shi *et al.*, 2020). The natural infection of pet cats, dogs and tigers via reverse zoonosis has also been reported (Newman, 2020; Sit *et al.*, 2020; Zhang *et al.*, 2020). Beyond the susceptibility of a given species to the virus, the ability for sustained animal-to-animal transmission is another important metric to assess. Ferrets have been demonstrated to be highly efficient at transmitting SARS-CoV-2 to uninfected animals via direct contact, and are also capable of airborne transmission, albeit less robustly (Richard *et al.*, 2020; Schlottau *et al.*, 2020; Shi *et al.*, 2020). The documented cases of SARS-CoV-2 infection in multiple mink farms in the Netherlands may provide an early indication of the possibility, and dangers, of reverse zoonosis (Enserink, 2020; Oreshkova *et al.*, 2020). The virus was observed to spread rapidly upon reaching a farm, and viral RNA was detected in airborne inhalable dust in the farms (Enserink, 2020; Oreshkova *et al.*, 2020). Two farm workers were also reported to have been infected (Enserink, 2020), demonstrating that newly infected animal populations can transmit SARS-CoV-2 back to humans.

Table 2. Susceptibility and transmission capability of different animal hosts to SARS-CoV-2.

Species	Natural Infection	Experimental Infection	Transmissible	Reference
Human (Homo sapiens)	Y	(–)	Y	(Guan et al., 2020)
Mouse (Mus musculus)	N	Y#	(–)	(Sun et al., 2020)
Rhesus macaque (Macaca mulatta)	N	Y	(–)	(Munster et al., 2020)
Crab-eating macaque (Macaca fascicularis)	N	Y	Y	(Rockx et al., 2020)
Dog (Canis lupus)	Y	Poor	N	(Sit et al., 2020) (Shi et al., 2020) (Almendros & Gascoigne, 2020)
Ferret (Mustela putorius furo)	N	Y	Y	(Shi et al., 2020) (Kim et al., 2020) (Schlottau et al., 2020)
Pig (Sus scrofa)	N	N	N	(Shi et al., 2020) (Schlottau et al., 2020)
Cat (Felis catus)	Y	Y	Y	(Shi et al., 2020)
Chicken (Gallus gallus)	N	N	N	(Shi et al., 2020) (Schlottau et al., 2020)
Duck (Anas platyrhynchos)	N	N	N	(Shi et al., 2020)
Egyptian fruit bat (Rousettus aegyptiacus)	N	Y	N	(Schlottau et al., 2020)
Tiger (Panthera tigris)	Y	N	(–)	(Wang et al., 2020)
Mink (Neovison vison?)	Y	N	(–)	(Oreshkova et al., 2020)
Syrian hamster (Mesocricetus auratus)	N	Y	Y	(Sia et al., 2020)

(–): Transmissibility has not been tested/reported.
#: Transgenic mice expressing human ACE2.

The reverse zoonosis potential of SARS-CoV-2 has two important implications. The first is the risk of transmission into livestock, which are commonly reared at high densities under intensive farming conditions around the globe. Thus far, pigs, duck and chickens have been reported to be not permissive to SARS-CoV-2 (Schlottau et al., 2020; Shi et al., 2020). At the time of writing, the susceptibility and transmission capability of SARS-CoV-2 in ruminants remains unknown, and is an important question to resolve, given the implications for global food security. The second is the concern for virus spillback from humans into Rhinolophus sp. or other permissive bat species, particularly in the Americas and Australia, geographical regions where SARSr-CoVs have not been detected previously (Wong et al., 2019). Reverse zoonosis could lead to the long-term establishment of this virus in these bat populations — the natural diversity of betacoronaviruses in bats, and frequent recombination events in coronaviruses, could also give rise to novel virus variants. Basic precautions to minimise the possibility of spillback include the use of appropriate personal protective equipment by farm-workers, zoological researchers and others who have frequent contact with animals (Gryseels et al., 2020). This also underscores the need for continued and active surveillance of virus populations in wild animals and key reservoir species globally, to rapidly inform public policy and healthcare decision-makers in the event such reverse zoonosis do occur.

Role of Serology for Future Animal Surveillance Studies

It is clear that there is still a long journey ahead for us to identify the true natural reservoir and potential intermediate host(s) for SARS-CoV-2, and the demonstrated ability for SARS-CoV-2 to transmit from human to animals will further complicate our investigation into the role of animals in the COVID-19 pandemic. Past studies have demonstrated that monitoring virus-specific antibodies is superior than detection of viral genetic materials, as antibodies generally last much longer than viral genetic material in animals (Li et al., 2005; Yob et al., 2001; Young et al., 1996). Sampling serum is also more reliable and uniform than other sampling approaches used for molecular detection, as the target tissues can vary from virus to virus (Barr *et al.*, 2015; Leroy *et al.*, 2005; Smith *et al.*, 2011). One challenge is to develop a serological test platform that can be used for different animals in a species-independent manner as an unknown number of animals will need to be sampled. In this context, our recently developed surrogate virus neutralisation test (sVNT) (Tan *et al.*, 2020) is ideal for filling this technological gap to facilitate large-scale animal surveillance. The sVNT platform is based on antibody mediated blocking of the RBD-ACE2 interaction, which mimics the virus neutralisation with the live virus and susceptible cell lines and can be conducted without relying on BSL3 containment. It can also work much faster, within an hour versus days required for live virus VNT.

Acknowledgement

The virus and bat research work conducted in our group is supported by grants from the National Research Foundation (NRF2012NRF-CRP001-056 and NRF2016NRF-NSFC002-013) and National Medical Research Council (STPRG-FY19-001 and COVID19RF-003), Singapore.

References

Ahn M, Anderson DE, Zhang Q *et al.* (2019) Dampened NLRP3-mediated inflammation in bats and implications for a special viral reservoir host. *Nat Microbiol* **4**(5):789–99. doi:10.1038/s41564-019-0371-3

Alagaili AN, Briese T, Mishra N *et al.* (2014) Middle East respiratory syndrome coronavirus infection in dromedary camels in Saudi Arabia. *mBio* **5**(2):e00884–00814.

Almendros A, Gascoigne E. (2020) Can companion animals become infected with Covid-19? *Veterinary Record* **186**:419.412–20. doi:10.1136/vr.m1322

Andersen KG, Rambaut A, Lipkin WI *et al.* (2020) The proximal origin of SARS-CoV-2. *Nat Med* **26**(4):450–52. doi:10.1038/s41591-020-0820-9

Barr J, Smith C, Smith I. (2015) Isolation of multiple novel paramyxoviruses from pteropid bat urine. *J Gen Virol* **96**(Pt 1):24–9. doi:10.1099/vir.0.068106-0

Brook CE, Dobson AP. (2015) Bats as "special" reservoirs for emerging zoonotic pathogens. *Trends Microbiol* **23**(3):172–80. doi:10.1016/j.tim.2014.12.004

Cagliani R, Forni D, Clerici M, Sironi M. (2020) Computational inference of selection underlying the evolution of the novel coronavirus, severe acute respiratory syndrome coronavirus. *J Virol* **94**(12). doi:10.1128/JVI.00411-20

Calisher CH, Childs JE, Field HE *et al.* (2006) Bats: Important reservoir hosts of emerging viruses. *Clin Microbiol Rev* **19**(3):531–45. Retrieved from http://www.ncbi.nlm.nih.gov/entrez/query.fcgi?cmd=Retrieve&db=PubMed&dopt=Citation&list_uids=16847084

Castillo AE, Parra B, Tapia P *et al.* (2020) Phylogenetic analysis of the first four SARS-CoV-2 cases in Chile. *J Med Virol.* doi:10.1002/jmv.25797

Chan JF, Zhang AJ, Yuan S *et al.* (2020) Simulation of the clinical and pathological manifestations of Coronavirus Disease 2019 (COVID-19) in golden Syrian hamster model: Implications for disease pathogenesis and transmissibility. *Clin Infect Dis.* doi:10.1093/cid/ciaa325

Cotten, M., Watson, S. J., Kellam, P., Al-Rabeeah, A. A., Makhdoom, H. Q., Assiri, A., Aal-Tawfiq, J., Alhakeem, R. F., Madani, H., AlRabiah, F. A., Hajjar, S. Al, Al-Nassir, W. N., Albarrak, A., Flemban, H., Balkhy, H. H., Alsubaie, S., Palser, A. L., Gall, A., Bashford-Rogers, R., … Memish, Z. A. (2013). Transmission and evolution of the Middle East respiratory syndrome coronavirus in Saudi Arabia: A descriptive genomic study. *The Lancet,* **382**(9909), 1993–2002. https://doi.org/10.1016/S0140-6736(13)61887-5

Coutard B, Valle C, de Lamballerie X *et al.* (2020) The spike glycoprotein of the new coronavirus 2019-nCoV contains a furin-like cleavage site absent in CoV of the same clade. *Antiviral Res* **176**:104742. doi:10.1016/j.antiviral.2020.104742

Cui J, Li F, Shi Z-L. (2019) Origin and evolution of pathogenic coronaviruses. *Nat Rev Microbiol* **17**(3):181–92.

Damas J, Hughes GM, Keough KC *et al.* (2020) Broad host range of SARS-CoV-2 predicted by comparative and structural analysis of ACE2 in vertebrates. bioRxiv.

Eden JS, Rockett R, Carter I *et al.* (2020) An emergent clade of SARS-CoV-2 linked to returned travellers from Iran. *Virus Evol* **6**(1):veaa027. doi:10.1093/ve/veaa027

Enserink M. (2020) Coronavirus rips through Dutch mink farms, triggering culls. In: American Association for the Advancement of Science.

Forster P, Forster L, Renfrew C, Forster M. (2020) Phylogenetic network analysis of SARS-CoV-2 genomes. *Proc Nat Acad Sci* USA **117**(17):9241–43. doi:10.1073/pnas.2004999117

Ge, XY, Li JL, Yang XL et al. (2013) Isolation and characterization of a bat SARS-like coronavirus that uses the ACE2 receptor. Nature 503:535–38. doi:10.1038/nature12711

Griffiths RC, Tavare S. (1994) Sampling theory for neutral alleles in a varying environment. Philos Trans R Soc Lond B Biol Sci 344(1310):403–10. doi:10.1098/rstb.1994.0079

Grubaugh ND, Petrone ME, Holmes EC. (2020) We shouldn't worry when a virus mutates during disease outbreaks. Nat Microbiol 5(4):529–30. doi:10.1038/s41564-020-0690-4

Gryseels S, De Bruyn L, Gyselings R et al. (2020) Risk of human-to-wildlife transmission of SARS-CoV-2. Preprint.

Guan WJ, Ni ZY, Hu Y et al. (2020) Clinical characteristics of coronavirus disease 2019 in China. N Eng J Med 382(18):1708–20. doi:10.1056/NEJMoa2002032

Guan Y, Zheng BJ, He YQ et al. (2003) Isolation and characterization of viruses related to the SARS coronavirus from animals in southern China. Science 302(5643):276–78. Retrieved from http://www.ncbi.nlm.nih.gov/entrez/query.fcgi?cmd=Retrieve&db=PubMed&dopt=Citation&list_uids=12958366

Hasegawa M, Kishino H, Yano T. (1985) Dating of the human-ape splitting by a molecular clock of mitochondrial DNA. J Mol Evol 22(2):160–74. doi:10.1007/BF02101694

Hoffmann M, Kleine-Weber H, Pohlmann S. (2020) A multibasic cleavage site in the spike protein of SARS-CoV-2 is essential for infection of human lung cells. Mol Cell 78(4): 779–84 e775. doi:10.1016/j.molcel.2020.04.022

Holmes EC, Dudas G, Rambaut A, Andersen KG. (2016) The evolution of Ebola virus: Insights from the 2013–2016 epidemic. Nature 538(7624):193–200. doi:10.1038/nature19790

Hu B, Zeng LP, Yang XL et al. (2017) Discovery of a rich gene pool of bat SARS-related coronaviruses provides new insights into the origin of SARS coronavirus. PLoS Pathog 13(11):e1006698. doi:10.1371/journal.ppat.1006698

Hu J, He C-L, Gao Q-Z et al. (2020) The D614G mutation of SARS-CoV-2 spike protein enhances viral infectivity and decreases neutralization sensitivity to individual convalescent sera. bioRxiv preprint. doi: https://doi.org/10.1101/2020.1106.1120.161323.

Huang C, Wang Y, Li X, Ren L et al. (2020) Clinical features of patients infected with 2019 novel coronavirus in Wuhan, China. Lancet 395(10223):497–506. doi:10.1016/S0140-6736(20)30183-5

Jones KE, Patel NG, Levy MA et al. (2008) Global trends in emerging infectious diseases. Nature 451(7181):990–93.

Kim YI, Kim SG, Kim SM et al. (2020) Infection and rapid transmission of SARS-CoV-2 in ferrets. Cell Host Microbe 27(5):704–09 e702. doi:10.1016/j.chom.2020.03.023

Lam TT, Jia N, Zhang YW et al. (2020) Identifying SARS-CoV-2-related coronaviruses in Malayan pangolins. Nature. doi:10.1038/s41586-020-2169-0

Lau SK, Woo PC, Li KS et al. (2005) Severe acute respiratory syndrome coronavirus-like virus in Chinese horseshoe bats. Proc Nat Acad Sci USA 102(39):14040–45. Retrieved from http://www.ncbi.nlm.nih.gov/entrez/query.fcgi?cmd=Retrieve&db=PubMed&dopt=Citation&list_uids=16169905

Leroy EM, Kumulungui B, Pourrut X et al. (2005) Fruit bats as reservoirs of Ebola virus. Nature 438(7068):575–76. Retrieved from http://www.ncbi.nlm.nih.gov/entrez/query.fcgi?cmd=Retrieve&db=PubMed&dopt=Citation&list_uids=16319873

Li W, Shi Z, Yu M et al. (2005) Bats are natural reservoirs of SARS-like coronaviruses. Science 310(5748):676–79.

Liu Y, Hu G, Wang Y et al. (2020) Functional and genetic analysis of viral receptor ACE2 orthologs reveals a broad potential host range of SARS-CoV-2. bioRxiv.

Lu J, du Plessis L, Liu Z et al. (2020a) Genomic epidemiology of SARS-CoV-2 in Guangdong Province, China. Cell 181(5):997–1003 e1009. doi:10.1016/j.cell.2020.04.023

Lu S, Zhao Y, Yu W et al. (2020b) Comparison of SARS-CoV-2 infections among 3 species of non-human primates. bioRxiv.

Millet JK, Whittaker GR. (2015) Host cell proteases: Critical determinants of coronavirus tropism and pathogenesis. Virus Res 202:120–34. doi:10.1016/j.virusres.2014.11.021

Munster VJ, Feldmann F, Williamson BN et al. (2020) Respiratory disease in rhesus macaques inoculated with SARS-CoV-2. Nature. doi:10.1038/s41586-020-2324-7

Nakamura T, Yamada KD, Tomii K, Katoh K. (2018) Parallelization of MAFFT for large-scale multiple sequence alignments. Bioinformatics 34(14):2490–92. doi:10.1093/bioinformatics/bty121

Newman A. (2020) First reported cases of SARS-CoV-2 infection in companion animals — New York, March–April 2020. Morb Mortal W Rep 69.

Normile D. (2020) Novel human virus. Pneumonia Cases Linked to Seafood Market in China Stir Concern.

O'Shea TJ, Cryan PM, Cunningham AA et al. (2014) Bat flight and zoonotic viruses. Emerg Infect Dis 20(5):741–45. doi:10.3201/eid2005.130539

Olival KJ, Hosseini PR, Zambrana-Torrelio C et al. (2017) Host and viral traits predict zoonotic spillover from mammals. *Nature* **546**(7660):646–50. doi:10.1038/nature22975

Oreshkova N, Molenaar R-J, Vreman S et al. (2020) SARS-CoV-2 infection in farmed minks, the Netherlands, April and May 2020. *Euro Surveill* **25**(23). doi:10.2807/1560-7917.ES.2020.25.23.2001005

Parrish CR, Holmes EC, Morens DM et al. (2008) Cross-species virus transmission and the emergence of new epidemic diseases. *Microbiol Mol Biol Rev* **72**(3):457–70. doi:10.1128/MMBR.00004-08

Pavlovich SS, Lovett SP, Koroleva G et al. (2018) The Egyptian rousette genome reveals unexpected features of bat antiviral immunity. *Cell* **173**(5):1098–110 e1018. doi:10.1016/j.cell.2018.03.070

Rambaut A. (2020) Phylodynamic Analysis. In *176 Genomes*: Virological.Org.

Richard M, Kok A, de Meulder D, Bestebroer TM. (2020) SARS-CoV-2 is transmitted via contact and via the air between ferrets. bioRxiv.

Rockx B, Kuiken T, Herfst S et al. (2020) Comparative pathogenesis of COVID-19, MERS, and SARS in a nonhuman primate model. *Science* **368**(6494):1012–15. doi:10.1126/science.abb7314

Schlottau K, Rissmann M, Graaf A et al. (2020) SARS-CoV-2 in fruit bats, ferrets, pigs, and chickens: An experimental transmission study. Lancet. doi:https://doi.org/10.1016/S2666-5247(20)30089-6).

Shang J, Ye G, Shi K et al. (2020). Structural basis of receptor recognition by SARS-CoV-2. *Nature* **581**(7807):221–24. doi:10.1038/s41586-020-2179-y

Sharp PM, Hahn BH. (2011) Origins of HIV and the AIDS pandemic. Cold Spring *Harb Perspect Med* **1**(1):a006841. doi:10.1101/cshperspect.a006841

Shi J, Wen Z, Zhong G et al. (2020) Susceptibility of ferrets, cats, dogs, and other domesticated animals to SARS-coronavirus 2. *Science* **368**(6494):1016–20. doi:10.1126/science.abb7015

Sia SF, Yan LM, Chin AWH et al. (2020) Pathogenesis and transmission of SARS-CoV-2 in golden hamsters. *Nature*. doi:10.1038/s41586-020-2342-5

Sit THC, Brackman CJ, Ip SM et al. (2020) Infection of dogs with SARS-CoV-2. *Nature*. doi:10.1038/s41586-020-2334-5

Smith I, Broos A, de Jong C et al. (2011) Identifying Hendra virus diversity in pteropid bats. *PLoS ONE* **6**(9):e25275. doi:10.1371/journal.pone.0025275 PONE-D-11-12458 [pii]

Su S, Wong G, Shi W et al. (2016) Epidemiology, genetic recombination, and pathogenesis of coronaviruses. *Trends Microbiol* **24**(6):490–502. doi:10.1016/j.tim.2016.03.003

Suchard MA, Lemey P, Baele G *et al.* (2018) Bayesian phylogenetic and phylody-namic data integration using BEAST 1.10. *Virus Evol* **4**(1):vey016. doi:10.1093/ve/vey016

Sun SH, Chen Q, Gu HJ *et al.* (2020) A mouse model of SARS-CoV-2 infection and pathogenesis. *Cell Host Microbe* **28**(1):124–33:e124. doi:10.1016/j.chom.2020.05.020

Tan CW, Chia WN, Qin X *et al.* (2020) A SARS-CoV-2 surrogate virus neutralization test based on antibody-mediated blockage of ACE2-spike protein-protein interaction. *Nat Biotechnol.* In press.

Tang L, Schulkins A, Chen C *et al.* (2020a) The SARS-CoV-2 spike protein D614G mutation shows increasing dominance and may confer a structural advantage to the furin cleavage domain. Preprint. doi: 10.20944/preprints202005.200407.v202001

Tang X, Wu C, Li X *et al.* (2020b) On the origin and continuing evolution of SARS-CoV-2. Nat Sci Rev **March**:1–12. https://doi.org/10.1093/nsr/nwaa1036.

Taubenberger JK, Kash JC. (2010) Influenza virus evolution, host adaptation, and pandemic formation. *Cell Host Microbe* **7**(6):440–51.

Taylor LH, Latham SM, Woolhouse ME. (2001) Risk factors for human disease emergence. *Philos Trans R Soc Lond B Biol Sci* **356**(1411):983–89.

Teeling EC, Vernes SC, Davalos LM *et al.* (2018) Bat biology, genomes, and the Bat1K project: To generate chromosome-level genomes for all living bat species. *Ann Rev Anim Biosci* **6**:23–46. doi:10.1146/annurev-animal-022516-022811

van Dorp L, Acman M, Richard D *et al.* (2020) Emergence of genomic diversity and recurrent mutations in SARS-CoV-2. *Infect Genet Evol* **83**:104351. doi:10.1016/j.meegid.2020.104351

Walls AC, Park YJ, Tortorici MA *et al.* (2020) Structure, function, and antigenicity of the SARS-CoV-2 spike glycoprotein. *Cell* **181**(2):281–92 e286. doi:10.1016/j.cell.2020.02.058

Wang L, Mitchell PK, Calle PP *et al.* (2020) Complete genome sequence of SARS-CoV-2 in a tiger from a U.S. zoological collection. *Microbiol Resour Announc* **9**(22). doi:10.1128/MRA.00468-20

Wang LF, Anderson DE. (2019) Viruses in bats and potential spillover to animals and humans. Curr Opin Virol **34**:79–89. doi:10.1016/j.coviro.2018.12.007

Wong ACP, Li X, Lau SKP, Woo PCY. (2019) Global epidemiology of bat coronaviruses. *Viruses* **11**(2). doi:10.3390/v11020174

Wong G, Bi YH, Wang QH *et al.* (2020) Zoonotic origins of human coronavirus 2019 (HCoV-19/SARS-CoV-2): Why is this work important? *Zool Res* **41**(3):213–19. doi:10.24272/j.issn.2095-8137.2020.031

Woo PC, Lau SK, Lam CS *et al.* (2012) Discovery of seven novel Mammalian and avian coronaviruses in the genus deltacoronavirus supports bat coronaviruses as the gene source of alphacoronavirus and betacoronavirus and avian coronaviruses as the gene source of gammacoronavirus and deltacoronavirus. *J Virol* **86**(7):3995–4008. doi:10.1128/JVI.06540-11

Xiao K, Zhai J, Feng Y *et al.* (2020) Isolation of SARS-CoV-2-related coronavirus from Malayan pangolins. *Nature.* doi:10.1038/s41586-020-2313-x

Yob JM, Field H, Rashdi AM *et al.* (2001) Nipah virus infection in bats (order Chiroptera) in peninsular Malaysia. *Emerg Infect Dis* **7**(3):439–41.

Young BE, Ong SWX, Kalimuddin S *et al.* (2020) Epidemiologic features and clinical course of patients infected with SARS-CoV-2 in Singapore. *JAMA.* doi:10.1001/jama.2020.3204

Young PL, Halpin K, Selleck PW *et al.* (1996) Serologic evidence for the presence in Pteropus bats of a paramyxovirus related to equine morbillivirus. *Emerg Infect Dis* **2**(3):239–40.

Yu WB, Tang GD, Zhang L, Corlett RT. (2020) Decoding the evolution and transmissions of the novel pneumonia coronavirus (SARS-CoV-2/HCoV-19) using whole genomic data. *Zool Res* **41**(3):247–57. doi:10.24272/j.issn.2095-8137.2020.022

Zehender G, Lai A, Bergna A *et al.* (2020) Genomic characterization and phylogenetic analysis of SARS-COV-2 in Italy. *J Med Virol.* doi:10.1002/jmv.25794

Zhang G, Cowled C, Shi Z *et al.* (2013) Comparative analysis of bat genomes provides insight into the evolution of flight and immunity. *Science* **339**(6118):456–60. doi:10.1126/science.1230835

Zhang Q, Zhang H, Huang K *et al.* (2020) SARS-CoV-2 neutralizing serum antibodies in cats: A serological investigation. bioRxiv.

Zhang YZ, Holmes EC. (2020) A Genomic perspective on the origin and emergence of SARS-CoV-2. *Cell* **181**(2):223–7. doi:10.1016/j.cell.2020.03.035

Zhao Z, Li H, Wu X *et al.* (2004) Moderate mutation rate in the SARS coronavirus genome and its implications. *BMC Evol Biol* **4**:21. doi:10.1186/1471-2148-4-21

Zhou H, Chen X, Hu T *et al.* (2020a) A novel bat coronavirus closely related to SARS-CoV-2 Contains natural insertions at the S1/S2 cleavage site of the spike protein. *Curr Biol* **30**(11):2196–2203 e2193. doi:10.1016/j.cub.2020.05.023

Zhou P, Yang XL, Wang XG *et al.* (2020) A pneumonia outbreak associated with a new coronavirus of probable bat origin. *Nature* **579**(7798):270–3. doi:10.1038/s41586-020-2012-7

Zhu N, Zhang D, Wang W *et al.* (2020) A novel coronavirus from patients with pneumonia in China, 2019. *N Eng J Med* **382**(8):727–33. doi:10.1056/NEJMoa2001017

4 The Global Perspective on the COVID-19 Pandemic

Darius LL Beh[1] and Dale A Fisher[2,3]

Introduction

On Dec 31, 2019, China reported a cluster of cases of pneumonia of unknown etiology with epidemiologic links to a seafood market in Wuhan. On Jan 5, 2020, after requesting additional information, the World Health Organization (WHO) issued a disease outbreak alert and reinforced standard surveillance of influenza and severe acute respiratory infections.[1] On Jan 30, the coronavirus disease 2019 (COVID-19) outbreak was declared a public health emergency of international concern (PHEIC)[2] and by Mar 11, with cases outside of China increasing 13-fold and the number of countries affected trebling, the Director-General of the WHO described the outbreak as a global pandemic.[3]

Global Epidemiologic Trends

COVID-19 spreads rapidly. From the initial epicenter in Wuhan, all 50 provinces in China were affected within a month. The first case outside of China was identified in Thailand on Jan 13.[4] Singapore was the next country affected with its first case identified on Jan 23.[5] By Jan 31, 106

[1] National Centre for Infectious Diseases
[2] Division of Infectious Diseases, National University Hospital, Singapore
[3] Yong Loo Lin School of Medicine, National University of Singapore

cases outside of China had been confirmed in 19 countries.[6] By Apr 1, it had spread to 201.[7]

An epicenter emerged in Lombardy in the North of Italy and quickly countries across Europe, most notably Spain experienced massive transmission overwhelming health service capacities. This resulted in massive nationwide lockdowns, where businesses were closed and the population instructed to remain at home. European countries peaked in late March at which time the epicenter moved to the United States. Europe and the US accounted for the vast majority of reported cases and deaths as of end April. By end May, South America had become the new epicenter of the pandemic, though by end August, Asia (excluding China) was contributing the largest proportion of daily confirmed cases, with a new epicenter over India (see Figure 1b).

Every region and every country has its own specific epidemiology and in one form or another experienced uncontrolled community transmission and subsequent lockdowns. New Zealand, several Australian states, and many Chinese provinces have shown the possibility of localized eradication

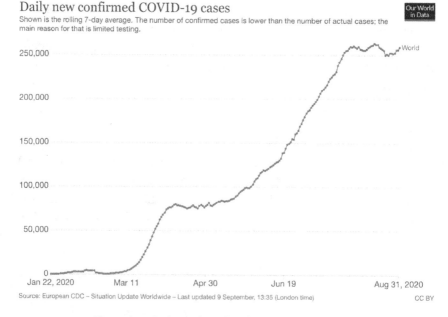

Daily new confirmed COVID-19 cases

Shown is the rolling 7-day average. The number of confirmed cases is lower than the number of actual cases; the main reason for that is limited testing.

Source: European CDC – Situation Update Worldwide – Last updated 9 September, 13:35 (London time)

CC BY

Figure 1a.   Daily number of confirmed COVID-19 cases.

Total confirmed COVID-19 cases

The number of confirmed cases is lower than the number of total cases. The main reason for this is limited testing.

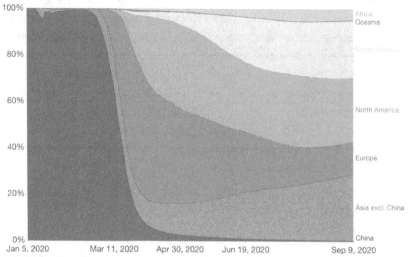

Figure 1b. Proportion of daily number of confirmed COVID-19 cases based on region.

Daily confirmed COVID-19 deaths

Limited testing and challenges in the attribution of the cause of death means that the number of confirmed deaths may not be an accurate count of the true number of deaths from COVID-19.

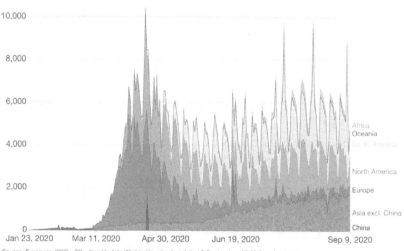

Figure 1c. Daily number of COVID-19 deaths based on region.

but the difficulties of maintaining this have been demonstrated with cases and clusters appearing sporadically. Other countries such as Vietnam, Thailand, Laos and Cambodia had strategies hinging on border controls but once breached significantly have needed various forms of lockdown to supplement a struggling public health response. Most parts of the world have chosen to target low case numbers relying on effective community engagement and a strong public health response to prevent or to rapidly shut down transmission chains. Other states, provinces and countries across the world bowed to political and economic pressures which saw a premature ending to lockdowns and a subsequent challenging resurgence of community transmission.

Response of the WHO

More than 7000 people with over 150 nationalities work for the Organization in 150 WHO country offices, with 6 regional offices overseen by its headquarters in Geneva, Switzerland.[8]

The WHO is one of 15 United Nations Agencies. It is committed to adhere to the principles set out in its constitution first drafted in 1946. Its role is to support the governments of almost 200 member states in their sovereign responsibility for the health of their people.

Since the start of the pandemic, the WHO helped countries prepare and respond, providing essential supplies and expertise. It developed training packages and where required, mobilized healthcare workers. It has also provided accurate information, clarified misinformation and supported research and development.

The WHO published the first COVID-19 Strategic Preparedness and Response Plan (SPRP) on Feb 3, 2020, with objectives for tackling the spread of disease at different levels[9]:

- Global — described the steps needed to rapidly establish international coordination to support countries to plan, finance and implement their response; provide a clear and transparent process to set research and innovation priorities, fast-track and scale-up research and development and ensure equitable availability of candidate therapeutics
- National — scale up preparedness and response operations

This framework is supported by the Operational Planning Guidelines to Support Country Preparedness and Response for countries to develop and update their COVID-19 national plans across 9 major pillars of COVID-19 preparedness and response.[10] These guidelines are designed to underpin the broader complementary strategies that make up the whole-of-UN, whole-of-government and whole-of-society approach to address parallel humanitarian and socioeconomic emergencies that may arise because of COVID-19.

The initial estimated resource envelope of this plan was US$675 million, of which US$61.5 million was intended for urgent preparedness and response activities. By May '20, WHO had received US$451 million from donors, including US$70 million from the recently set up COVID-19 Solidarity Response Fund. The Fund was created at the request of the WHO by the United Nations Foundation (UNF) in partnership with the Swiss Philanthropy Foundation (SPF), and aims to diversify funding by enabling private corporations, the general public, foundations and other organizations to directly support the COVID-19 response led by the WHO. By the same time, the Solidarity Fund allocated US$75 million to WHO for the supply chain facility to purchase essential commodities, US$10 million to UNICEF for work at a national level, US$10 million to the Coalition for Epidemic Preparedness Innovations (CEPI) for vaccine development, and US$20 million to the World Food Programme (WFP) for commodity logistics and transportation. The COVID-19 Partners Platform was launched to be an enabling tool for all countries, donors and contributors to jointly plan resource needs, allocate resources and identify gaps. The Partners Platform features real-time tracking and allows access to the Supply Portal for countries to request and receive globally sourced COVID-19 critical supplies through the UN COVID-19 Supply Chain System (CSCS).[11]

The UN Development Coordination Office (UNDCO) led the development of a UN framework to help countries address the multidimensional socio-economic aspect of the crisis using a wide and flexible range of support modalities.[12] The unique scale of the crisis has required the WHO to reach beyond member states and member state groupings, such as African Union, ASEAN, the EU, the G7, the G20, the G12 donors, to include partnerships with the World Economic Forum (WEF), International Chamber of Commerce (ICC), the International Organization of Employers, the UN Global Compact.

The WHO was quick to establish a global surveillance system gathering data from member states which is stored and shared in a central database. This data, along with daily case and death counts from 212 countries, territories, and areas, are analyzed and presented globally to inform and support high-level strategic decision making. Tailored analyses are produced regularly on request for member states in addition to a global situation report, including multiple Disease Outbreak News bulletins related to the spread of COVID-19.

On Apr 20, WHO, the International Telecommunication Union (ITU) with support from UNICEF announced a partnership to work with telecommunication companies to provide COVID-19 related health education via text messages to reach billions of people that are currently unable to obtain the information available on the internet.[13] To counter the "infodemic" — the overabundance of information of varied quality and accuracy, the WHO developed the WHO Information Network for Epidemics (EPI-WIN).[14] EPI-WIN translates new science into evidence-based messaging and information products. By end April, EPI-WIN had published more than 130 FAQs, videos and animations, infographics and messaging, and "myth busters". WHO, in collaboration with UNICEF and IFRC have developed a "COVID-19 Global Response — Risk Communication and Community Engagement Strategy for all partners" guidance document, to help member states navigate essential risk communication with their communities.[15]

Diagnostic testing has been a key COVID-19 response strategy — test, isolate and trace to interrupt chains of transmission. Tracking of cases also allows governments to identify clusters and estimate the burden of disease so as to advise on the appropriate measures. In early February, WHO announced that they were shipping 250,000 diagnostic tests to 70 laboratories around the world.[16] WHO reference laboratories established across the six WHO regions expanded to include 24 laboratories with expertise in virology, diagnostics, sequencing, and viral culture by end April.[17] These supported countries that did not have testing capacity or needed validation of their initial test results while building capacity. In addition, surveillance testing for COVID-19 was initiated in clinics caring for patients with influenza-like illness (ILI) as part of the Global Influenza Surveillance and Response System. Genetic sequence data provided through the GISAID influenza genetic sequence database has provided insights to tracking and tracing the COVID-19 lineages and variants. By end April, almost 16,000 SARS-CoV-2 genome sequences had been shared through the GISAID database.

The WHO has also provided technical expertise, guidance and support. By early April, 1.2 million people had enrolled in the OpenWHO training platform, which has COVID-19-specific courses available in 43 languages.[18] Technical missions supported countries including Ethiopia, São Tomé and Príncipe, Tajikistan, Papua New Guinea and Timor-Leste. WHO and GOARN partners are working to facilitate online ArcGIS, a geographic information system (GIS) software training to build and improve the operational capacity of partners. Direct technical assistance is facilitated through GOARN, with experts from 27 partner institutions being deployed to provide support to countries directly or through remote assistance. Go-Data is a database to support contact tracing and other outbreak response needs. It was developed by WHO in collaboration with partners in GOARN. As of September, there were approximately 60 Go.Data projects worldwide. Access to emergency health workforce capacity is coordinated through the over 100 Emergency Medical Teams (EMTs). As of end April, 19 EMTs have been internationally deployed, with another 36 EMTs supporting national operations.

At the intial outset, with no vaccines or curative treatments, an emergency mechanism to coordinate research and development efforts on a global scale was needed. On Feb 11-12, the WHO convened the Global Research Forum, to engage a diverse group of policy makers, researchers, public health experts, non-governmental organizations, brought together with funders and the private sector.[19] Using the WHO R&D Blueprint as its basis, the Forum developed an initial COVID-19 Global Research Roadmap,[20] which would later take shape as the Access to COVID-19 Tools (ACT) Accelerator.[21] On May 4, donors delivered, pledging US$8 billion to the Coronavirus Global Response Initiative, and on Jun 4, Global Vaccine Summit raised $8.8 billion from 32 donor governments and 12 foundations, corporations and organizations to immunize 300 million children and support the global fight against COVID-19.[22] The WHO rapidly published guidance on how to accelerate vaccine development and guidance on vaccine development prioritization.

Table 1. Summary of key WHO responses to the COVID-19 pandemic; the first 6 months.

Date	Helping Countries Prepare and Respond
Jan 28	• WHO meets with China's leadership to collaborate on containment, studies on severity and transmissibility, and continued sharing of data and biologic material; plans to send international experts and reconvene the International Health Regulations (IHR 2005) Emergency Committee[187]
Feb 5	• Launch of $675 million **Strategic Preparedness and Response Plan (SPRP)** to rapidly establish international coordination and operational support, scale up country readiness and response operations and accelerate priority research and innovation[9]
Feb 9	• WHO deploy an advance team for the WHO-China Joint Mission[4]
Feb 12	• Launch of **COVID-19 Partners Platform**
Mar 1	• Announcement of **COVID-19 Solidarity Response Fund** to raise money from a wide range of donors support the work of the WHO and partners to help countries respond to the COVID-19 pandemic[188] • Release of US$15 million from the **UN Central Emergency Response Fund (CERF)** to help vulnerable countries contain the spread of COVID-19
Mar 26	• WHO Director-General calls on **G20 to Fight, Unite, and Ignite** against COVID-19; G20 committed to support and further strengthen WHO's mandate in coordinating the response, and called for full funding of WHO's Strategic Preparedness and Response Plan[189]
Mar 30	• WHO releases guidelines to help countries maintain essential health services during the COVID-19 pandemic[190]
Apr 3	• **WHO and UNICEF to partner** on pandemic response through COVID-19 Solidarity Response Fund[191]
April 18	• Global Citizen organized **'One World: Together at home' Global Special curated by Lady Gaga** in support of the WHO raised almost $128 million for the COVID-19 Solidarity Response Fund[192,193]
Apr 30	• Third meeting of the **International Health Regulations (2005) Emergency Committee** regarding the outbreak of coronavirus disease (COVID-19)[194]
May 11	• WHO Director-General informal briefing to **United Nations Economic and Social Council (ECOSOC)** on 'Joining Forces: Effective Policy Solutions for Covid-19 Response'[195]
Date	Provision of Essential Supplies
Feb 2	• First dispatch of **RT-PCR lab diagnostic kits** shipped to WHO Regional Offices[4]
Feb 27	• Release of interim guidance on the **Rational use of personal protective equipment (PPE)** and strategies to optimize the availability of PPE *(revised on Apr 6, 2020)*[196]

Table 1. *(Continued)*

Date	Provision of Essential Supplies
Mar 3	• WHO supplied half a million sets of PPE to 47 countries, and calls on industry and governments to increase manufacturing by 40% to meet rising global demand[197] • Works with governments, industry and the **Pandemic Supply Chain Network** to boost production and secure allocations for critically affected and at-risk countries[198]
Mar 30	• **COVID-19 Essential Supplies Forecasting (ESTF)** Tool developed to help health providers to forecast needs of essential supplies during a pandemic *(revised Apr 24)*[199]
Jun 4	• The **Gavi COVAX Advance Market Commitment (AMC)** is launched at the Global Vaccine Summit, an innovative financing instrument of the **COVID-19 Vaccines Global Access Facility (COVAX Facility)** to secure access to timely and sufficient supply of vaccines for developing countries.[200]

Date	Training and Mobilization of Healthcare Workers/Expertise
Jan 25	• **OpenWHO** launches first educational modules on COVID-19: "Emerging respiratory viruses, including nCoV: methods for detection, prevention, response and control"[201]

Date	Global Health Education
Mar 23	• WHO in conjunction with **FIFA** launch awareness campaign to tackle COVID-19: Pass the message to kick out coronavirus" campaign promotes five key steps for people to follow to protect their health in line with WHO guidance[202]
Mar 20	• **WHO Health Alert** is launched, offering instant and accurate information about COVID-19 on WhatsApp
Apr 20	• **ITU-WHO Joint Statement: Unleashing information technology** to provide COVID-19 health education via text messaging[13]
May 13	• Launch of the **WHO Academy (WHOA) app** designed to support health workers during COVID-19, and the WHO Info app designed to inform the general public *(information previously available on WHO websites)*[203]

Date	Research and Development
Feb 6	• WHO convenes a **Global Research and Innovation Forum** to mobilize international action in response to the new coronavirus (2019-nCoV) in line with the WHO R&D Blueprint[204] • Creation of a **WHO COVID-19 database**, updated daily from searches of bibliographic databases, hand searching, and the addition of other expert-referred scientific articles[205]
Feb 13	• WHO's Digital Solutions Unit convenes a roundtable of 30 companies in Silicon Valley to help build support for WHO to keep people safe and informed about COVID-19

(Continued)

Table 1.   *(Continued)*

Date	Research and Development
Mar 6	• WHO publishes the **Global Research Roadmap** developed by the working groups of the Research Forum
Apr 24	• Heads of state and global health leaders pledge to work towards equitable global access based on an unprecedented level of partnership at a virtual event, co-hosted by the WHO[206] • Launched a Global Collaboration to accelerate the development, production and equitable **Access to new COVID-19 Tools (ACT)** including diagnostics, therapeutics and vaccines[21] • On Jun 26, ACT-Accelerator published its consolidated investment case, calling for $31.3 billion over the next 12 months
Jun 3	• As of 3 June 2020, more than 3500 patients in 400 hospitals have been recruited in 35 countries to participate in the **Solidarity Trial**[207]

The ACT-Accelerator was a ground breaking global collaboration to accelerate development, production, and equitable access to COVID-19 tests, treatments and vaccines. It brought together leaders of governments, global health organizations, businesses and philanthropic groups in a united response against COVID-19.[23]

On Mar 18, 2020 to accelerate research of therapeutics, the WHO launched Solidarity — a large international multicenter trial to compare four treatment options against standard care — remdesivir; lopinavir-ritonavir; lopinavir-ritonavir with interferon beta-1a; and chloroquine or hydroxychloroquine. On Jun 4, WHO accepted the recommendation from the Solidarity Trial's International Steering Committee to discontinue the trial's hydroxychloroquine and lopinavir/ritonavir arms.[24] On July 27, WHO published an initial draft landscape of COVID-19 vaccine candidates including 25 vaccines under clinical evaluation.[25] This was subsequently expanded to include 42 vaccines undergoing clinical trials and 151 vaccine candidates in pre-clinical evaluation.[25]

Criticisms of the WHO

Too Trusting of China

WHO has been accused (mostly by the United States but also other countries) of having been unduly influenced by, or too trusting of China in its response to the COVID-19 pandemic.[26] Critics have argued that the WHO should have sought greater transparency from China, should have declared a PHEIC sooner, and should have restricted trade and travel to and from China.[27] On Apr 14, 2020 US President Donald Trump, speaking at the White House said the "WHO's reliance on China's disclosures likely caused a 20-fold increase in cases worldwide". On Apr 15, the US President cut funding to the WHO[28] and on May 29, he announced at a press conference that he would 'terminate' the United States' relationship with the organization.[29] At present the WHO is already grossly underfunded. It's two-year budget for 2020-2021 of $4.8 billion is roughly the budget of a large hospital in the US and $2 billion less than the annual budget of the Center for Disease Prevention and Control (CDC).[30]

A review of the timeline however shows that on Jan 14, 2020, WHO tweeted that "Preliminary investigations conducted by the Chinese authorities have found no clear evidence of human-to-human transmission of the novel #coronavirus".[31] The tweet has been used as evidence of the WHO's stand, however it is worth noting that earlier that day at a press conference in Geneva, it was also stated that human-to-human transmission may be occurring on a limited scale as seen with other respiratory pathogens.[32]

China informed the WHO on Jan 12 that no additional cases had been detected since Jan 3, and with the closure of the Wuhan Seafood market on Jan 1, this suggested that infections were associated with zoonotic transmission and exposure to the market.[33]

The WHO is an evidence-based organization and can only report on the information that they have. Within the 2005 International Health Regulations (IHR), it is the obligation of member states to promptly notify the WHO of novel events, however this framework does not give the WHO the authority to compel them to do so or inspect a member state and conduct its own investigations without the authorization of the state in question.[34] Even if a state violates the IHR, the WHO has no formal enforcement mechanism.

Experts from the WHO from its China and Western Pacific regional offices proceeded to conduct a brief field visit from Jan 20-21 to Wuhan[35] and on Jan 22, the WHO mission issued a statement saying there was evidence of human-human transmission but more investigation was needed to understand the full extent.[36] Human-to-human transmission would eventually be confirmed with a publication in the *Lancet* on Jan 24.[37]

Travel Restrictions

The WHO initially advised against the application of travel and trade restrictions to countries experiencing COVID-19, citing evidence that restricting the movement of people or goods during a public health emergency is ineffective, may divert resources from other interventions and cause economic harm.[38]

It subsequently endorsed travel restrictions, but only at the beginning of an outbreak citing evidence that it may provide countries time to prepare for their response.[39]

Mask Wearing

The WHO initially recommended the use of masks for those sick or if taking care of a person who is suspected of having COVID-19. It was not recommended for the well and asymptomatic general public.

That position was adopted by countries such as the US, UK, much of Europe, Australia, New Zealand, India, South Africa and Singapore. Other measures such as handwashing and social distancing was emphasized instead with the understanding that masks needed to be conserved for healthcare workers. However, on Apr 3, both the US (following CDC recommendations) and Singapore changed their advice on mask wearing and recommended the use of masks in the community. As of Apr 14, Singapore took a further step to make mask wearing in public mandatory.[40] Changes in the recommendations were based on evolving epidemiologic data confirming that cases of pre-symptomatic transmission of SARS-CoV-2 had been confirmed.[41] Other studies comparing the temporal dynamics of viral shedding with the epidemiologic parameters of the disease have concluded that the infectious period begins 2.3 days before and peaks 0.7 days before the onset of symptoms.[42]

On Jun 5, the WHO updated their advice on community mask wearing in light of evolving evidence and in line with the advice from its technical advisory group.[43] Governments were advised to encourage the public to wear masks "where there is widespread transmission and physical distancing is difficult".[44]

Country-Specific Case Studies

China

Upon the detection of a cluster of pneumonia cases of unknown etiology in Wuhan in Dec 2019, the Communist Party of China Central Committee and the State Council launched a national emergency response. A Central Leadership Group for Epidemic Response and the Joint Prevention and Control Mechanism of the State Council was established.[45]

During the early stage of the outbreak, the main strategy focused on preventing the exportation of cases from Wuhan. Wet markets, such as the Huanan Seafood Market were closed on Jan 1, 2020.[46] During the second stage of the outbreak, the main strategy was to reduce the intensity of the epidemic and to slow down the spread of infection. On Jan 23, with 571 confirmed cases and 17 deaths, Wuhan, a city of 11 million people was placed under a strict lockdown. This proved later to become a template for future responses globally. Spring Festival holidays were extended, public transportation shut down, and travel restrictions implemented to reduce the movement of people. Strict physical distancing was implemented and wearing of face masks in public mandated. Public health messaging included information about the epidemic and control measures. Public risk communications and health education was strengthened; allocation of medical supplies was coordinated and the Wuhan leadership had 2 new hospitals built in just 10 days.[36,47]

By Feb 10, when the advance team of the WHO-China Joint Mission began its work, China was reporting over 2000 new cases daily. Two weeks later at the completion of the full mission (16-24 February 2020), that number had dropped to just over 400 cases/day.[48] Their report praised China for its "bold approach to contain the rapid spread of this new respiratory pathogen" but it warned that this virus had potential for "major health, social and economic impact" and that the world was "not prepared in capacity or mindset".[45]

The third stage of the outbreak in China focused on reducing clusters of cases. For Wuhan and priority areas of Hubei, concrete steps were taken to decrease transmission by testing, isolating and treating all patients. Not all cities and regions were managed the same way, but "a risk-based pre-vention and control approach was adopted with differentiated measures for different regions".[45] New technologies were applied such as the use of big data and artificial intelligence to enhance contact tracing.

Despite these measures, dealing with a new emerging infectious disease, with many unknowns, such as transmission dynamics, pattern of disease and disease severity, hospitals in Wuhan were overwhelmed.[49] This may partly explain the higher case fatality rate reported in Wuhan compared to other parts of China (5.8% vs 0.7%).[45] Daily confirmed cases peaked in early February with about 3800 reported daily. However, by early March, it had decreased to less than 200 with the total confirmed cases reaching a plateau of just over 80,000 cases, with around 4000 deaths.[50]

At the height of China's lockdowns, 500 million people were affected by some form of travel and movement restrictions. In Wuhan after 11 weeks of intensely enforced lockdown on Apr 8, people could leave their houses.[51]

In late May, after having no new cases for weeks in Wuhan, a cluster of cases was found in a residential compound, sparking fears of a second wave. China responded by conducting a city-wide screening of 11 million people in just 2 weeks — confirming and isolating 300 cases.[52]

China clearly has zero tolerance for COVID-19 with an unstated eradication strategy. On Jun 11, a cluster of cases was identified at Xinfadi wet market in Beijing[53] prompting millions of tests and placing hundreds of thousands in lockdown. The cluster was limited to under 400 cases but demonstrated what would appear to be the standard by which China would respond to cases in the future. Over the ensuing year China maintained its zero tolerance for cases. With clusters continuing to emerge, often in market places, focused lockdowns with mass testing were maintained as the recurrent strategy. The increased transmissibility of Delta represented a challenge to the success of this approach.

United States

The first case of COVID-19 in the US was identified on Jan 20, 2020 in Washington State in a returning traveler from Wuhan, China, with no contact with the Huanan Seafood Market.[54] With growing indications that at least limited human-to-human transmission was occurring,[55] the CDC activated the Emergency Operations Centre to handle the response to the outbreak.[56] They announced their own RT-PCR test and raised the travel alert notice for travelers from Wuhan. Public health screenings were implemented first in airports at San Francisco, New York and Los Angeles, followed by Atlanta and Chicago.[57] With a second travel-related case identified on Jan 23 in a Chicago resident who had returned from Wuhan 10 days prior,[58] the CDC recommended that travelers avoid all non-essential travel to Wuhan. By Jan 27, this was extended to include the rest of China.[59] On Jan 29, the CDC issued a 14-day federal quarantine for 195 Americans returning from Wuhan[60], and similar measures were implemented officially for all travelers from China from Feb 2. However, the CDC's "decades-old notification system, riddled with errors and duplicate records made tracking passengers exceedingly difficult".[61]

It was not until Feb 3, that the CDC began shipping COVID-19 test kits to public health laboratories, and by Feb 6, just 90 kits had been distributed.[62] However, on Feb 12 the CDC had to issue a recall as the kits were unreliable.[63] This would later be attributed to laboratory contamination causing false positives in the control samples.[61] On Feb 16, the CDC and FDA met to discuss solutions to the testing problem, such as removing the component of the test thought to be the cause.[64] On Feb 18 the CDC warned laboratories against using tests without an "emergency use authorization". As of Feb 20, of the more than 100 public health laboratories in the US, only three were capable of testing. Despite this, based on a *Washington Post* investigation, the FDA continued to place bureaucratic hurdles to laboratories seeking approval for tests they had developed.[64] As of Feb 22, with 78,572 confirmed cases globally, only 258 tests were being run per day — with 15 cases within the US being identified in total. [62]

In keeping with poor capacity, the US CDC continued to instruct state health authorities to only test patients with a travel history to China.[62] On Feb 19, a California woman with flu-like symptoms was admitted to the University of California-Davis Medical Center, who sought immediate COVID-19 testing by the CDC. This was denied as the patient did not fit the testing criteria. It was not until Feb 23 that the CDC ordered testing, and on Feb 27, they announced that this was the first confirmed case of community spread in the US, together with an announcement that the flawed test kits were rectified and that their testing criteria would be expanded to include any person suspected of having COVID-19 by a clinician.[65]

Testing capacity however remained very limited, leading the FDA to implement a new policy to take advantage of tests developed by commercial, reference, and clinical laboratories nationwide as a push to expand capacity.[66]

Three cases highlight the early sustained community transmission: two deaths on Feb 6 and 17 in California identified though post-mortem tissue specimens and an unidentified passenger or crew member aboard a Pacific cruise ship that left San Francisco on Feb 11, whose genomic sequence of viruses has been traced back to the Washington clade. Cryptic circulation of the virus was occurring by early February likely resulting from the importation of a single lineage of virus from China in late January, followed by several importations from Europe.[67]

On Mar 2, the US administration shifted strategy from containment to mitigation in keeping with influenza pandemic plans.[68] The WHO had stated that containment was an important strategy to mitigate and that it should not be an all or nothing policy. Indeed, there had been a fear that countries could adopt an inappropriate influenza mitigation strategy for this novel coronavirus. In the subsequent weeks, despite expanding testing over 60-fold, the number of confirmed cases increased 600-fold, and on Mar 13, with 2179 confirmed cases and 49 deaths, the US President Donald Trump declared a National Emergency in order to access billions in more funding to address the epidemic.[62]

By Mar 16, with every state having declared an emergency, the White House announced a voluntary program called "15 Days To Slow The Spread," a nationwide effort to decrease transmissions of COVID-19 through the implementation of social distancing — two weeks after key members of the White House coronavirus task force believed the administration should begin advocating such measures.[62,69] Following the first lockdown in the San Francisco area on Mar 16, many states followed with their own lockdown measures.

On Mar 27, the Association for Professionals in Infection Control and Epidemiology (APIC) released the results of a national survey showing dire shortages of personal protective equipment (PPE) across the US.[70] Almost half (48%) of the US-based infection preventionist members reported that their healthcare facilities were already or almost out of respirators used in caring for patients with COVID-19. The Defense Production Act allows the federal government to direct US companies to prioritize production of certain goods in emergencies, such as PPE. Although the administration had discussed the Act as early as mid-January, the law was not enacted until the end of March.[62] With questions about Federal leadership and the coordination of supply procurement, Grassroots organizations GetUsPPE and Project N95 collaborated to establish a Demand Data Hub Partnership — a single online platform for healthcare facilities to report their PPE needs, improve the understanding of PPE demand and serve to provide equitable distribution of PPE.[71] Based on their data from end April, for those providers requesting PPE through their platform, 20% had run out of N95 respirators already, 41% had less than a week's supply, 28% had a 1–2 week's supply; and only 11% had supplies expected to last for more than 2 weeks.[71-73]

Job losses surged and Congress passed the $2 trillion CARES Act to offer some financial relief to the public and businesses.

As of May 31, there were 1.77 million confirmed cases and 103,781 deaths in the US.[50] The Presidential Statements throughout reflected a disconnect, prioritization of the economy and an underestimation of the severity of the COVID-19 pandemic.[50] With the crisis deepening, tensions between President Trump and CDC increased with concerns of perceived leaks, marked by public condemnations on Twitter and a tendency to dismiss findings from scientists.[61] The first failure was implementation of widespread testing. The second was a delay in travel restrictions from Europe which may have bought some time to better prepare. The third was problems with the public health record-keeping system and the CDC's use of antiquated systems to manage data. For this, it has been described as "risk-averse, perfectionist and ill-suited to improvising in a quickly evolving crisis" and "increasingly bureaucratic, weighed down by indescribable, burdensome hierarchy".[61] The constitutional structure of the US places the primary responsibility of public health with the states. Lacking a strong federal leadership to guide a unified response, the US quickly fulfilled the WHO's prediction of being ill prepared in capacity and mindset and became the new epicenter of the COVID-19 pandemic.[74]

There are many lessons to be learned, much of which was captured by Dr Mike Ryan, the Executive Director of the WHO Emergencies Program during a press conference on Mar 13: "Be fast. Have no regrets. You must be the first mover. The virus will always get you if you don't move quickly. If you need to be right before you move, you will never win."[75]

United Kingdom

The UK confirmed the first two cases of COVID-19 on Jan 31, 2020 in two Chinese nationals in York; neither of whom met the testing criteria at the time.[76] The day before, the four UK Chief Medical Officers (CMO) agreed to escalate planning and preparation in case of a more widespread outbreak and increased the risk level from low to moderate.[77] The third case was identified on Feb 6, in a returning traveler from Singapore who spread the virus to 11 others on a ski trip to the French Alps before returning home.[78] Following this, the UK expanded its self-isolation policy and clinical case definition for returning travelers with flu-like symptoms to include 8 countries/regions in Asia, in addition to China.[79]

Nine days prior to confirming its first case, on Jan 22, the UK government convened the first meeting of its scientific advisory group for emergencies (SAGE). Preliminary estimates of the basic reproduction number (R_0) then was 2.6–3.5, and a 60% reduction in transmissions was predicted to be needed in order to control the spread — i.e. potentially a lockdown.[80] The UK had a head start on testing: hundreds of people were tested for every early case and this was complemented by comprehensive contact tracing early on. However, the UK failed to expand testing capacity sufficiently in the month of February.[50]

On Feb 10, the UK introduced the Health Protection (Coronavirus) Regulations 2020 (superseded by the Coronavirus Act 2020) to impose restrictions on individuals at risk of spreading COVID-19. This gave health professionals the power to detain patients with COVID-19 for screening and assessment, or to isolate them for a period of time, and also allow police to detain people suspected of having the virus.[81] On Feb 26, with 7,132 people tested and 13 positive, the UK Health Secretary issued a statement describing the 4-phase plan to respond to COVID-19: contain, delay, research, mitigate. So as to free up National Health Service (NHS) resources, an isolation facility at Heathrow airport was also set up for international passengers who needed testing. Travelers returning from affected areas were also recommended to self-isolate and call NHS 111, even if they had no symptoms.[82]

On Mar 3, the UK government published their COVID-19 action plan detailing actions taken to date and the next steps of their 4-phase plan, with a focus then on containment.[83] During the press briefing, Prime Minister Boris Johnson reassured the public to go about their business as the country was extremely well prepared and told reporters that he continues to shake hands.[84]

During early March, cases began increasing exponentially and testing was no longer able to keep up with the need (see Figure 3a).[50] By the second week of March, compared to Germany's 20,000 tests per day, the UK was averaging under 2,000 tests per day.[85] On Mar 12, the UK moved from containment to a "delay" phase, and announced a controversial move to cease tracing and testing the contacts of coronavirus patients. The risk of COVID-19 to the UK was escalated from 'moderate' to 'high' and the first self-isolation measures were introduced for people with symptoms, regardless of travel history. The Prime Minister changed tack, saying "this is the worst public health crisis for a generation", but emphasized that the government would not close schools[86] — however, just 6 days later, school closures would be announced.[87] During this time, one of the busier weekends in the sporting calendar continued with hundreds of thousands gathering for a horse racing carnival. Despite a lack of guidance, rugby and soccer associations acted and canceled matches.[88]

Although the new focus was to "delay" the spread, new social distancing measures were only announced 4 days later, on Mar 16, at a first daily press briefing with the Prime Minister, CMO, Chris Whitty and Chief Scientific Adviser, Patrick Vallance. In addition, two new measures were introduced to delay the spread of the disease (self-isolation for people with two key symptoms and their households, and a cessation of non-essential travel).[89] During this press conference, Vallance mentioned the government's

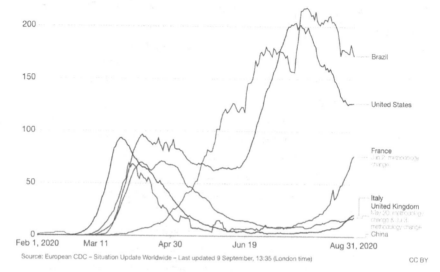

Daily new confirmed COVID-19 cases per million people

Shown is the rolling 7-day average. The number of confirmed cases is lower than the number of actual cases; the main reason for that is limited testing.

Source: European CDC – Situation Update Worldwide – Last updated 9 September, 13:35 (London time)

CC BY

Figure 2a. Daily number of new COVID-19 cases in the US, UK, France, Italy, Brazil and China.

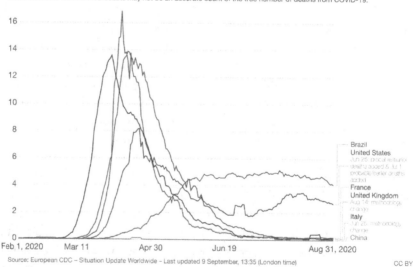

Daily new confirmed COVID-19 deaths per million people

Shown is the rolling 7-day average. Limited testing and challenges in the attribution of the cause of death means that the number of confirmed deaths may not be an accurate count of the true number of deaths from COVID-19.

Source: European CDC – Situation Update Worldwide – Last updated 9 September, 13:35 (London time)

CC BY

Figure 2b. Daily number of new COVID-19 deaths in the US, UK, France, Italy, Brazil and China.

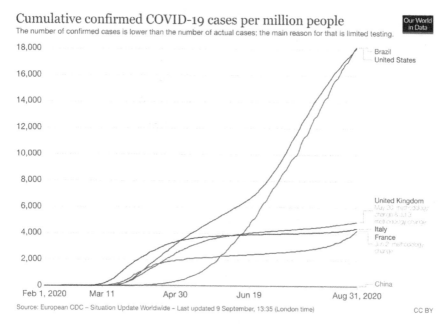

Figure 2c. Total COVID-19 cases in the US, UK, France, Italy, Brazil and China.

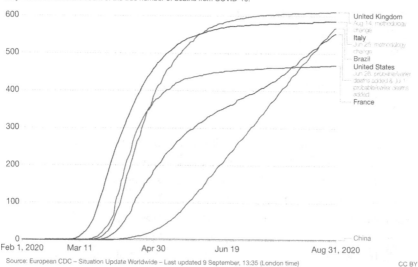

Figure 2d. Total COVID-19 deaths the US, UK, France, Italy, Brazil and China.

Case fatality rate of the ongoing COVID-19 pandemic
The Case Fatality Rate (CFR) is the ratio between confirmed deaths and confirmed cases. During an outbreak of a
pandemic the CFR is a poor measure of the mortality risk of the disease. We explain this in detail at
OurWorldInData.org/Coronavirus

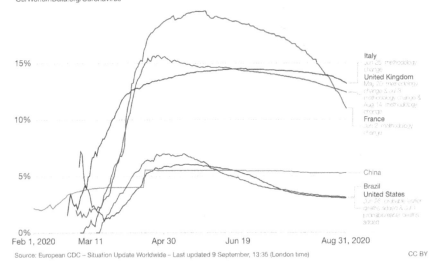

Source: European CDC – Situation Update Worldwide – Last updated 9 September, 13:35 (London time)   CC BY

Figure 2e.   Case fatality rate in the US, UK, France, Italy, Brazil and China.

long-term goal was for the UK to develop "some kind of herd immunity".
Almost immediately, the supposed plan came under heavy criticism — herd
immunity is typically achieved through mass vaccination, and not through
exposure to a deadly virus.[88,90] Though never official policy but when said
at the time of a policy vacuum, it sent a confusing message.[85] Since then,
the Health Secretary stated that the goal was like other countries (to flatten
the curve) and herd immunity may be achieved as a consequence of this,
but it was not the aim.[90]

   With regards to imposing strong measures earlier, the UK government's
stand was that it was important to impose the measures at the right time
and guided by scientific evidence to ensure they coincided with the peak
of the disease, however with doubts in the scientific community, a call was
made for the evidence to be made public.[91] On the same day, a modelling
paper was published suggesting there could be around 250,000 deaths
in the UK if milder 'mitigation' measures were pursued.[92] Meanwhile, on
Mar 8, Northern Italy went into lockdown — one that was extended to all

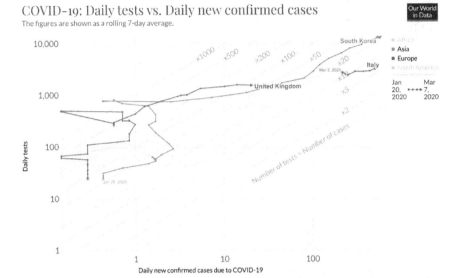

Figure 3a.   Daily tests vs daily new confirmed cases — UK vs South Korea and Italy.

of Italy the next day and on Mar 14 and 17, Spain and France followed suit respectively.

On Mar 19, the UK government committed to ramping up testing from 5000 a day to 10-25,000 with the eventual aim of 250,000.[93] On Mar 20, pubs and restaurants were ordered to shut as part of a move to close entertainment, hospitality and indoor leisure premises.[94] This came 9 days after modelers had delivered new projections to the government — time the government took to deliberate how and when a lockdown should be introduced.[95] The UK was very late to deliver its definitive strategy.

The total number of NHS hospital beds has more than halved over the past 30 years. Whilst this trend has been observed in other advanced healthcare systems (to a lesser degree), the UK has fewer acute and critical care beds relative to its population.[96,97] These shortfalls of the healthcare system were already known in 2016, revealed by Operation Cygnus, a simulation exercise to study the impact that a pandemic influenza would have on the UK. The exercise showed that the pandemic would cause the

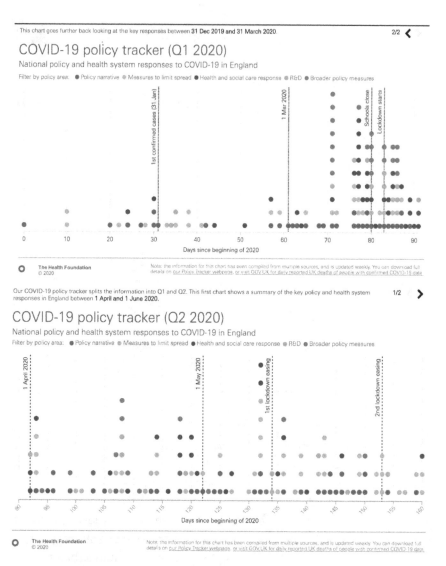

Figure 3b.   National policy and health system responses to COVID-19 in England.[105,106]

country's health system to collapse from a lack of resources and highlighted a lack of ventilators. The list of recommendations to address these deficiencies was never implemented.[98]

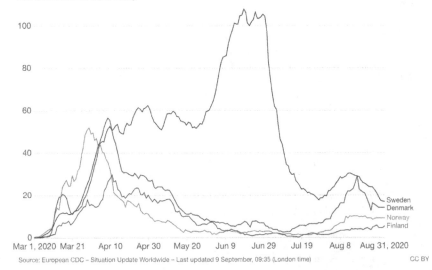

Figure 4a. Daily new confirmed COVID-19 cases per million people for Sweden compared to Denmark, Norway and Finland.

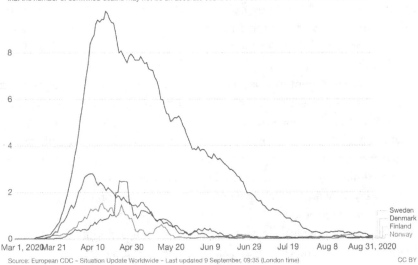

Figure 4b. Daily new confirmed COVID-19 deaths per million people for Sweden compared to Denmark, Norway and Finland.

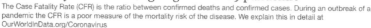

Case fatality rate of the ongoing COVID-19 pandemic

The Case Fatality Rate (CFR) is the ratio between confirmed deaths and confirmed cases. During an outbreak of a pandemic the CFR is a poor measure of the mortality risk of the disease. We explain this in detail at OurWorldInData.org/Coronavirus

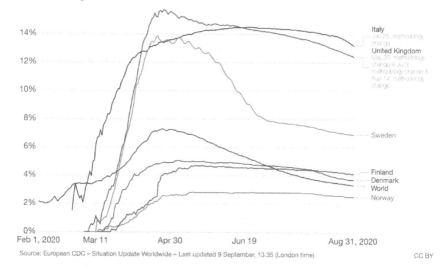

Figure 4c. Case fatality rate in the Nordic countries compared to Italy and UK.

On Apr 3, the Health Secretary claimed that the government was "working round the clock to deliver essential deliveries of PPE across the whole NHS, social care, key public services, and in all 4 nations of the UK".[99] On May 15, it was reported that more than 100 healthcare workers had contacted WhistleblowersUK raising concerns about COVID-19 and PPE.[100]

The government has been criticized for being late to recognize the need to replenish stockpiles of PPE and ventilators that had dwindled during the years of austerity cuts. Shortfalls were meant to be filled by "just in time" contracts, however many were with Chinese manufacturers who faced increasing demand from their own country's health service. The British Healthcare Trades Association (BHTA) was ready to help supply PPE in February and March however it was only on Apr 1 that it's offer of support was accepted.[80]

The shortages led doctors to protest with the slogan "Doctors not Martyrs".[101] Thousands of doctors also commenced legal action demanding the government launch a public inquiry to investigate the failure to provide

NHS and care staff with adequate PPE. As of May 20, 200 NHS and care workers had died after becoming infected with COVID-19.[102]

As of May 31, the UK had over 270,000 confirmed cases, and over 45,000 deaths — one of the highest globally and per capita.[50,103] 32.5% of all COVID-19 deaths had been in care homes.[103] The Prime Minister having only attended his first cabinet meeting on COVID-19 on Mar 2, 5 weeks after the first meeting on the issue, was criticized for a lack of oversight on managing the COVID-19 response.[80] The delay in increasing testing, in limiting large gatherings, and in issuing a lockdown all drew criticism.[95] The lack of travel bans was especially important with a preliminary analysis of genomic sequences suggesting that the UK epidemic was driven by a very large number of importations due to inbound international travel from Italy in mid-Feb, followed by Spain and France in early March.[104]

After many months without imposing travel restrictions, the UK government on Jun 8 introduced a blanket 14-day self-isolation commitment on all incoming travellers.

At the end of April, the Prime Minister promised the public a 'comprehensive plan' for easing social distancing measures and by early May the publication of the 'COVID-19 recovery strategy' outlined the steps to lifting lockdown restrictions. This began on May 13 by allowing those who could not work from home to return to work and to allow people to take part in 'unlimited' outdoor exercise. During this time, the government worked to address shortages in PPE, increase testing and improve reporting standards.[105,106] The UK's epidemic curve plateaued in May and showed signs of a downward trend by mid-May, with the daily number of confirmed cases decreasing from approximately 5000 per day in late April to about 1500 per day by end May. The daily deaths had also decreased in tandem.[50]

Sweden

Sweden took a different approach to combat COVID-19. While there were some restrictions such as voluntary social distancing, no gatherings above 50, and since Apr 1, 2020, a visiting ban on the country's care homes for the elderly, the general approach was less severe than in other countries.[107,108] People continued to commute to work, restaurants remained open (with measures to ensure distancing), and so did primary schools.[107] Sweden did not mandate mask wearing in public, citing a lack of evidence supporting this recommendation.[107]

The architect of the strategy, Anders Tegnell, is an infectious disease physician and since 2013, served as a state epidemiologist at Sweden's Public Health Agency, an independent body whose expert recommendations the government follows.[109]

Swedish laws on communicable diseases focuses on a citizen's individual responsibility to take measures to prevent the spread of disease.[109] This concept relies on a bedrock of trust between the government and its people, and its citizens have taken this responsibility seriously; practicing social distancing, with the elderly isolated and families mostly staying home. Apple mobility trends showed a 50% drop by mid-March[110].

The approach has drawn sharp critics, especially with regards to the slow response to the threat in elderly care facilities, which contributed significantly to the higher number of deaths compared to its Nordic neighbors.[109] As such, they responded by prioritizing testing for vulnerable groups.[108]

While the daily number of confirmed cases plateaued in Sweden at around 50-60 cases per million per day, those in Denmark, Norway and Finland continued on a downward trajectory at less than 10 cases per million per day (see Figure 2a). As for total confirmed deaths, as of May 31, Sweden recorded 4395 deaths, compared to 571, 236 and 316 deaths from Denmark, Norway and Finland respectively.[50]

Sweden has affirmed multiple times that the strategy is not intended to achieve herd immunity but like most countries, to flatten the curve as much as possible so as to avoid overwhelming the healthcare system.[111] However, Tegnell has also mentioned before that whilst lockdowns do seem to work to reduce cases significantly, many countries end their lockdowns with low levels of immunity and dealing with this long-term can be difficult.[107] Despite this softer approach, based on a seroepidemiologic survey published in May 2020 only 7.3% of adults 20–65 years of age in Stockholm had antibodies to SARS-CoV-2, with the rate lower in other age groups and other parts of Sweden.[112]

Economists estimated that Sweden's GDP would drop 6.5% in 2020, about the same as the US and Germany, but better than the 9-10% declines estimated for Finland and Denmark, all of which had lockdowns.[113] As such some countries emerging from lockdown have looked to Sweden's model with a hope to balance the needs of the economy with a desire to keep people healthy — both physically and mentally. However, Sweden's Nordic neighbors have not shared these views. By mid-June as European countries reopened their borders to EU tourists, due to Sweden's looser containment strategy and higher mortality rate, Denmark, Norway and Finland kept their borders closed to Sweden.

Though still higher than its Nordic neighbors, as of August the number of daily cases and daily deaths reduced significantly from its peak in June,[50] and in early September they reported their lowest PCR test positivity rate to date — 1.2%.[114]

New Zealand

While most countries took measures to 'flatten the curve', New Zealand was more ambitious, and aimed to eliminate COVID-19 completely.[115] And for much time, their strategy had been largely successful, drawing admiration around the world. Although, eradication had problems in creating a community expectation and increasing the challenges to opening borders. In contrast, most other countries have preferred low numbers with rapid identification of cases, shutting down of small transmission chains and avoiding super-spreader events.

Early on, while COVID-19 was still mainly in China, and against WHO advice at the time, New Zealand banned entry to foreign travellers from China starting from Feb 3, 2020, in order to reduce the possibility of an outbreak in New Zealand and to allow time for the health system to prepare.[116] On Feb 28, New Zealand reported its first confirmed case, in a New Zealand citizen who had recently visited Iran, returning via Bali, Indonesia.[117] At that time, border restrictions were in place for anyone who had visited mainland China or Iran in the past 14 days. By Mar 19, at 28 confirmed COVID-19 cases (all imported/linked), New Zealand closed all borders and entry ports to all non-residents, while returning citizens and residents were required to self-isolate.[118] This later became two weeks of supervised quarantine from Apr 9 onwards.[119]

On Mar 21 they introduced a country-wide alert level system, similar to the existing fire warning systems with four levels — 1 being the least risk of infection and 4 the highest.[120] At the time of the announcement the country was at level 2. On Mar 23, with an additional 2 suspected cases of community spread and at only 103 confirmed cases, they moved to level 3.[121] By Mar 25, they announced a move to level 4 and introduced a strict nationwide lockdown that was projected to continue for 4 weeks,[122] and was later extended a further week.

Citizens isolated at home, except those providing essential services, and were only allowed to leave to exercise in their neighborhood and visit those in another residence as part of a shared bubble arrangement. Bars, restaurants and any places of public gathering were closed, and all non-essential businesses were shut. Supermarkets and pharmacies remained open, though only 1 family member was permitted entry at a time. Physical distancing was encouraged, and breaches of the above were policed.[123]

Quarantines and lockdown measures were paired with widespread testing and contact tracing. As of May 31, New Zealand had performed over 280,000 tests, with a peak of almost 8000 tests per day in early May, and about 240 tests for each confirmed case.[50,124] By comparison, South Korea which used innovative approaches to scale up testing had performed about 80 tests for each confirmed case.[50] Geography also played a part — New Zealand is relatively isolated, is able to close entry points to the country and has a low population density.[125]

Prime Minister Jacinda Ardern's crisis leadership skills and risk communication has attracted international attention and praise. It took courage and leadership to reach beyond containment and aim for elimination and during this crisis, she has united the country with firm, humane and consistent messaging.[126,127]

On Apr 27, New Zealand announced that they were winning the battle against COVID-19, with no widespread, undetected community transmission.[128] They entered alert level 2 on May 14, while maintaining physical distancing in public and for private gatherings with more than 10 people.[129] This was later raised on May 25 to 100 people.[130] Despite easing lockdown restrictions, New Zealand did not report any locally acquired cases since May 22 with their total confirmed cases remaining at 1,504 and 24 deaths.[124] The country removed all remaining restrictions except border controls on June 8, moving back to Level 1.

On Aug 11, after 102 days free of COVID-19, New Zealand confirmed 4 cases in the community, in one family acquired from an unknown source, and with this, the country reinstated Level 3 lockdown restrictions.[131] Through Aug, 77 community cases would be linked to the August cluster and placed in isolation facilities.[132]

Vietnam

Vietnam reported the first case of COVID-19 on Jan 23, 2020.[133] A week later, a national steering committee was established to coordinate Vietnam's government strategy.[134] Travelers from Wuhan, China, received additional screening, and visas for Chinese tourists were no longer issued from Jan 30. Flights to and from China were suspended on Feb 1, and trains canceled shortly after. Starting in early February, international arrivals from countries affected by COVID-19 were placed in large government-run quarantine centers.[135]

On Feb 13, provincial leaders declared quarantine measures in Son Loi, a commune in Vinh Phuc, a northern province about an hour from Hanoi. Patients and their close contacts were quarantined in camps for at least 14 days and community-wide screening was initiated at first signs of community spread.[135,136] On Mar 6, Vietnam experienced a second wave of imported cases from those returning from Europe, UK and the US.[135] On May 1, a hundred days into the outbreak, Vietnam had confirmed just 270 cases despite extensive testing.[137] By end July, Vietnam had gone more than 3 months without recording any new cases of local transmission, and there were no deaths attributed to COVID-19.[138]

However, an unexplained outbreak occurred in the coastal city of Danang, affecting hospitals with elderly patients. It spread to 15 cities and provinces before coming under control.[51] By Aug 31, Vietnam had reported 1040 cases and 32 deaths.[50]

Part of Vietnam's successful management of the COVID-19 pandemic has been attributed to investments in public health infrastructure following the SARS outbreak. During 2000–2016 Vietnam's public health expenditure per capita increased at a rate of 9 percent per year, and with that, key health indicators such as infant and maternal mortality decreased significantly.[139,140] Vietnam also established a national emergency operations center in 2013 and four regional centers in 2016.[141] These are staffed by alumni from the Field Epidemiology Training Program, which was established in 2007 with support from WHO and the US CDC.[142,143] Their purpose is to conduct exercises to train key stakeholders in the government for outbreaks. Since 2016, Vietnam's Ministry of Health has been able to track epidemiologic data across the country in real time — supported by web-based systems and requirements for hospitals to report notifiable diseases to a central database within 24hrs.[144,145]

Case detection and contact tracing have been key components of Vietnam's containment strategy. In late January, the Ministry of Science and Technology hosted a meeting with virologists to encourage the development of diagnostic tests. By early February, publicly funded institutions had locally developed four COVID-19 tests using in-house versions of the WHO protocol and validated by the Ministry of Defense. Private companies such as Viet A and Thai Duong supported the manufacturing capacity to mass produce test kits cheaply. Vietnam expanded testing capacity from just two sites in late January to 120 by May.[135]

With low case numbers, the country decided on a strategy of testing to identify clusters. When community transmission was detected, the government responded with contact tracing, commune-level lockdowns and further local testing to ensure no cases were missed. At one point, Vietnam had performed more tests per confirmed case than any other country in the world (see Figure 5b).[135]

Vietnam's contact tracing strategy stands out as uniquely comprehensive — it is based on tracing degrees of contact from the index case and applying different degrees of isolation for the different levels of contact (as shown in Figure 6).[135] This approach to testing or quarantining suspect cases based on epidemiologic risk and not symptoms is worth mentioning. With evidence highlighting that the infectious period begins two days before symptoms, this approach had the benefit of rapidly tracking and quarantining contacts before they became infectious.[42] The high proportion of asymptomatic cases identified (43%) suggests this approach can limit community transmission early.[146]

Vietnam implemented targeted lockdowns in suspected hot spots based on evolving epidemiologic data and also entered a nationwide lockdown on Apr 1, lasting up to 21 days in some areas.[135] While leaders in many countries downplayed the threat of COVID-19, the Vietnamese government communicated clearly via text messaging, social media, remade a well-known pop song into a handwashing public service announcement now known as "Ghen Co Vy" and even organized a dance challenge on Tik Tok.[135,147] On Apr 14, Vietnam passed a decree to levy fines against those who spread online falsehoods, and though this has generated opposition from Amnesty International, 93% of Vietnamese people believe their government has responded "very" or "somewhat" well.[148] Vietnam was one of the few South East Asian economies forecasted to report GDP growth in 2020.[149]

India

As of Aug 31, 2020, in terms of total coronavirus cases, India had surpassed Brazil, coming in second only to the US.[150] With over 75,000 cases a day, it also had the fastest growing coronavirus outbreak of any country and became the new epicenter of the pandemic.[151]

On Jan 30, India reported its first case of COVID-19 in Kerala, with two others on Feb 3 from students who had returned from Wuhan.[152] Apart from these, no significant rise in transmissions was observed in February. India implemented surveillance as early as Jan 17 and introduced travel advisories and restrictions with efforts to repatriate and quarantine Indian nationals arriving from abroad.[153] On Feb 4, India canceled existing visas for Chinese nationals and foreigners who had visited China in the two weeks prior.[154]

In March, transmissions increased as a number of travelers from affected countries returned to India. As of Mar 28, 909 cases and 19 deaths in 27 states and union territories had been reported.[155] With cases rising, on Mar 25, Prime Minister Narendra Modi exercised executive powers under the Disaster Management Act of 2005 and issued a lockdown of the country. All incoming international flights were suspended, and

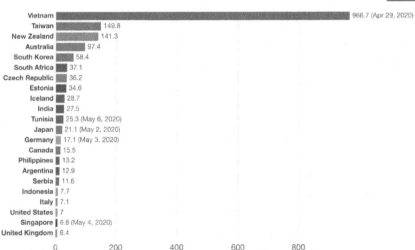

Total COVID-19 tests for each confirmed case, Jun 1, 2020

New Zealand	243.5 (May 30, 2020)
Australia	202.4 (May 31, 2020)
Taiwan	163.6 (May 31, 2020)
South Korea	80.1
Denmark	45.3
Norway	29.2 (May 29, 2020)
Russia	26.9
Germany	22.2 (May 24, 2020)
India	20.5 (May 31, 2020)
Canada	18.6
Japan	17.3
Italy	16.8
Spain	10.7 (May 28, 2020)
United States	9.6 (May 31, 2020)
Indonesia	8.8
United Kingdom	8.5 (May 22, 2020)
Sweden	7.2 (May 24, 2020)
Singapore	6.9 (May 25, 2020)
Brazil	1.1 (May 29, 2020)

Source: Testing data from official sources collated by Our World in Data, confirmed cases from ECDC   OurWorldInData.org/coronavirus · CC BY
Note: Comparisons of testing data across countries are affected by differences in the way the data are reported. Details can be found at our Testing Dataset page.

Figure 5a. Testing rates for various countries (as of Jun 1, 2020).

Total COVID-19 tests for each confirmed case, May 5, 2020

Vietnam	966.7 (Apr 29, 2020)
Taiwan	149.8
New Zealand	141.3
Australia	97.4
South Korea	58.4
South Africa	37.1
Czech Republic	36.2
Estonia	34.6
Iceland	28.7
India	27.5
Tunisia	25.3 (May 6, 2020)
Japan	21.1 (May 2, 2020)
Germany	17.1 (May 3, 2020)
Canada	15.5
Philippines	13.2
Argentina	12.9
Serbia	11.6
Indonesia	7.7
Italy	7.1
United States	7
Singapore	6.8 (May 4, 2020)
United Kingdom	6.4

Source: Testing data from official sources collated by Our World in Data, confirmed cases from ECDC   OurWorldInData.org/coronavirus · CC BY
Note: Comparisons of testing data across countries are affected by differences in the way the data are reported. Details can be found at our Testing Dataset page.

Figure 5b. Testing rates for various countries (as of May 5, 2020).

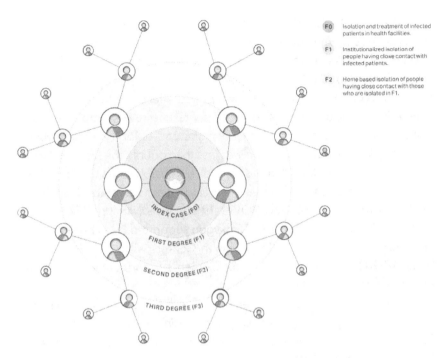

Figure 6. Third degree contact tracing in Vietnam.

interstate movement restricted.[155] Initially forecasted to last 21 days, the population of over 1.3 billion people were only given a 4 hour notice. It would subsequently be extended to 10 weeks. Whilst effective in countries such as China, the lockdown in India was criticized for failing to take into account the specific socio-economic contexts of an average Indian workers life — around 95% of workers are informal, with no social protection. The lockdown deprived these workers of paid employment, generating severe economic distress in groups already living on the margin of subsistence. With little public assistance, it is likely this amplified vulnerabilities to all diseases, including COVID-19. Provisions to address food insecurity were only implemented 45 days after lockdown. A third of the urban population also live in dense and crowded conditions with no access to clean access and soap. As such the stay-at-home policy meant physical distancing norms could not be adhered to, and frequent handwashing impractical for most.[156]

The aim of a lockdown is to *contain* an outbreak temporarily while allowing governments time to expand, train and deploy the public health force. However, very limited funds were made available for immediate public health expenditure (less than 0.04%) and with the exception of Kerala, many states did not use the lockdown period effectively to test, trace and quarantine to reduce transmission.[156] Low testing rates hampered India's ability to manage the outbreak: toward the end of lockdown, on May 3, the testing rate of 758 per million was less than double the rate just before lockdown.[156,157] On May 31, there were over 180,000 cases and over 5000 deaths.[157] Despite shortfalls, health infrastructure was ramped up during the lockdown. 930 dedicated COVID-19 hospitals with 158,747 isolation beds, 20,355 ICU beds and 69,076 oxygen supported beds became available. 2362 dedicated COVID-19 Health Centers with 132,593 Isolation beds; 10,903 ICU beds and 45,562 oxygen supported beds were also operationalized.[158]

Once lockdown measures were eased, with the loss of jobs, millions of migrant workers returned to their villages, spreading the virus to rural areas.[151] State governments in India played a key role managing and coordinating the health system, and as in other countries, the response has varied in different communities. More than half of all COVID-19 cases during this time were concentrated in three states: Maharashtra, Tamil Nadu, and Karnataka, which could not be accounted for by higher testing rates.[153]

With a cumulative number of 3.6 million confirmed cases and 65,000 deaths as of Aug 31, India's test positivity rate remained high at just under 8%.[50] Sero-surveillance surveys of populations in Mumbai slums, Pune and Delhi found a seropositivity of 57%, 50% and 23% respectively,[159] suggesting then that the true scale of the outbreak and deaths in India may indeed be much higher than reported.

Other Countries

Countries across the globe have adopted different approaches or implemented similar strategies in a unique style. There is much to learn by studying these varied responses.

For example, South Korea's early success was credited to its efforts in ramping up testing to about 10,000 per day and pursuing rigorous

Daily new confirmed COVID-19 cases

Shown is the rolling 7-day average. The number of confirmed cases is lower than the number of actual cases; the main reason for that is limited testing.

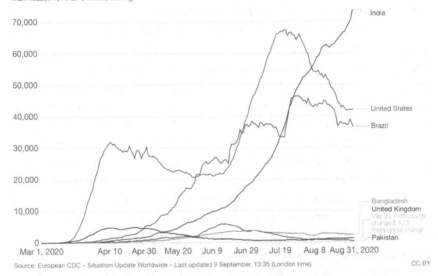

Figure 7a. Daily new confirmed COVID-19 cases in India compared to other neighboring countries, the US, UK and Brazil.

Daily new confirmed COVID-19 deaths

Shown is the rolling 7-day average. Limited testing and challenges in the attribution of the cause of death means that the number of confirmed deaths may not be an accurate count of the true number of deaths from COVID-19.

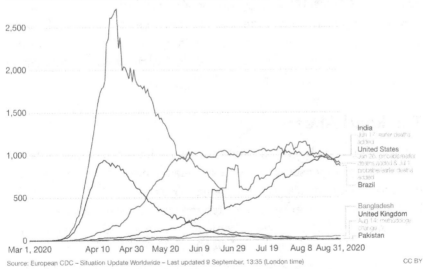

Figure 7b. Daily new confirmed COVID-19 deaths in India compared to other neighboring countries, the US, UK and Brazil.

contact tracing for all confirmed cases plus instituting a quarantine for their contacts. As such, cases dropped from 600/day in February to 100/day in April, whilst tests/day increased, showing the success of the strategy.[50]

Japan took a pragmatic approach to COVID-19 that has been largely successful. Though they had limited testing capabilities early and limited resources, they took a cluster-based approach to identify and contain the spread of infections. COVID-19 was also quickly designated an infectious disease by law requiring hospitalization of all positive patients. Authorities promoted the avoidance of closed spaces, crowded places, and close-contact settings. While the government could not order the closure of businesses due to political pressure, they instead requested many shops, bars, and restaurants to close out of a sense of social responsibility. Many complied to avoid risking their reputation and being blamed for spreading disease out, which may have had more significant commercial and financial implications. The cultural practices of mask-wearing and cleanliness has also been attributed to their initial success in managing COVID-19.[160,161]

President Bolsonaro was credited as being the greatest threat to Brazil's fight against COVID-19. He actively dismissed COVID-19 as a threat and discouraged physical distancing and lockdown implemented by state government and city mayors, sacking the health minister who criticized his actions.[162] When Brazil became the epicenter of the disease, it took down cumulative COVID-19 data, purportedly to hide its soaring death toll, only reporting daily figures. President Bolsonaro threatened exit from the WHO after it warned of the dangers of lifting lockdowns before slowing the spread of disease. At which point, Brazil had the third highest number of the deaths outside of the US & UK.[163,164]

The Road Ahead

In this chapter, we hoped to capture some of the defining moments: the important early measures, the styles of leadership and the strategies of many countries particularly during the first six months of the pandemic. Following the first wave, experts predicted repetitive smaller waves, a fall peak or a slow burn.[165] These have all come true in some way, shape and form.

As of Jul 1, 2021, China recorded 91,780 infections and 4,636 deaths. In contrast, the US with a population one-quarter that of China, recorded

33.6 million cases with roughly 604,000 deaths.[166] Over the past year, China has experienced small, scattered clusters of cases and overall, has been able to keep these outbreaks under control through a combination of isolated lockdowns, mass testing, digital contact tracing,[167] mandatory quarantine and adherence to social distancing and hygiene measures.[166] In the US, a combination of state economic re-openings, mass gatherings,[168] political rallies,[169] air travel over the holidays and a lack of universal mask wearing have all been cited to have contributed to the most devastating wave of infections over the fall and winter months of 2020.[170] In the United Kingdom, despite increasing restrictions over the winter months, the country experienced a surge in infections and reached a record number of 55,892 daily cases on Dec 31, 2020.[171] This surge would later be attributed to a new, more transmissible variant of SARS-CoV-2 known as B.1.1.7 or later, the alpha variant.[172] Despite being early to approve and start mass vaccination with the Pfizer/BioNTech vaccine, due to cases overwhelming the health system, the UK had to enter into its third lockdown on Jan 5, 2021.[173,174] Since then, the UK and US have both made significant progress with mass vaccination and as of Jul 1, 2021, almost 50% of their population had received 2 doses of the COVID-19 vaccine and were considered fully immunized. On Jul 19, the UK ended lockdowns and restrictions with the declaration of "freedom day", a moment felt by many to be premature and extreme. At the same time, China had fully vaccinated 16% of their population.[50] Vaccine inequity remains a pressing issue, with the overwhelming majority of vaccine doses being administered in high income countries. This has led the WHO to warn countries of the consequences of a 'two-track pandemic'.[175]

Sweden continued its open approach and has one of the highest infection rates in western Europe. This has led to protests for the government to change their national approach: to test and trace more, recommend face masks and enforce regulations about social distancing and ventilation.[176] New Zealand's elimination strategy has stood out amongst others, with the defining addition of instituting early lockdowns in response low level community spread. So far, this strategy has been effective at keeping daily cases in the single digits and going for periods without any community transmission, earning them the title of being COVID-19 free. This is despite relatively lower rates of vaccination (6.6% as of Jun 15, 2021).[50] This strategy has relied on strict border controls, crippling it's tourism industry resulting in significant economic impact.

Vietnam was held up as one of the gold standards for its COVID-19 response and in spite of low vaccination rates, was able to keep their daily cases under 10 for many months. However, a surge in cases in late May 2021 illustrated that with the emergence of more transmissible variants of concern and because border controls are vulnerable to infection control breaches, they have since decided to rely on significant social restrictions until the vaccination rate is adequate to enable its non-pharmaceutical public health interventions.[177]

India appeared to be controlling transmission as early as Feb 2021, however frequent large-scale events drawing millions of unmasked individuals combined with a more contagious delta variant contributed to a second wave that would dwarf the first.[178] As of May, India became the epicenter of the pandemic and at its peak officially recorded over 400,000 daily cases and close to 5000 daily deaths.[50] In the wake of India's COVID-19 crisis, a 'black fungus' epidemic followed with thousands of cases of invasive mucormycosis reported.[179]

By Oct 2020, the WHO Solidarity trial had recruited 12,000 patients in 500 participating hospitals across 30 countries, and published an interim report showing that 4 repurposed antiviral drugs had little or no effect on mortality and the need for mechanical ventilation in hospitalized patients with COVID-19.[180] As of July 23, 2021, COVAX, the vaccine pillar ACT Accelerator shipped over 138 million vaccines to 136 participating locations.[181] Despite these achievements and its continued effort, the WHO became an easy target to blame for the mishandling of the pandemic. Its response to such political attacks was to remind countries "not to politicize this virus".[182] Nevertheless, with the majority of funding arising from three sources, it is important for the WHO to diversify, and if member states want the WHO to be smaller, more focused and one with more authority, it is ultimately up to them to propose the necessary legislative changes and pass a vote. Yet, with all its limitations and challenges, the WHO is still the most suitable organization to convene a global conference and tackle the COVID-19 pandemic.

Some countries have emerged from lockdown, apparently free of COVID-19, only to discover a new cluster of cases either from previously undetected community spread or from reintroductions. Others are still trying to figure out how to safely reopen their economies and their borders. From each country's response, there are lessons to be learned. While there are some strategies that have been more effective than others, there isn't a universal strategy that can or should be adopted by all countries. Some studies have attempted to compare the strategies adopted by various countries in order to weigh the efficacy of non-pharmacologic interventions and their timing respective to the local epidemic.[106,183]

How COVID-19 has played out on a global stage draws stark similarities to a contemporary board game inspired by the SARS outbreak and aptly named "Pandemic". As members of "the CDC", each with unique roles, players must cooperate and move across the globe to stop the spread of four diseases. As its game designer puts it: "No single player can win this alone. We all need to play to our strengths, balance short-term threats against long-term goals and make sacrifices for the common good. If we can communicate, coordinate and cooperate effectively we might better overcome this uncaring, relentless and frightening opponent."[184]

COVID-19 has been able to find its way into even the most remote communities[185] and form clusters of outbreaks in population dense facilities, such as migrant worker dormitories, hospitals, meat processing plants, churches, nursing homes and prisons. Even after this time the virus will remain endemic causing cases, small clusters and will continue to take lives. COVID-19 has exposed many weaknesses in each country's government organizations, public health systems, and overall pandemic preparedness. In a post COVID-19 pandemic world mankind has an opportunity to learn and grow but whether we do, and how we do, is a chapter in this saga that is yet to be written.

References

1. Pneumonia of unknown cause — China [press release]. World Health Organization (WHO), Jan 5 2020.

2. Statement on the second meeting of the International Health Regulations (2005) Emergency Committee regarding the outbreak of novel coronavirus (2019-nCoV) [press release]. World Health Organization (WHO), Jan 30 2020.

3. WHO Director-General's opening remarks at the media briefing on COVID-19 — 11 March 2020 [press release]. World Health Organization (WHO), Mar 11 2020.

4. Timeline of WHO's response to COVID-19 [press release]. Jun 29 2020.

5. Confirmed Imported Case of Novel Coronavirus Infection in Singapore; Multi-Ministry Taskforce Ramps Up Precautionary Measures [press release]. Jan 23 2020.

6. WHO. Novel Coronavirus(2019-nCoV) Situation Report — 11. World Health Organization; Jan 31 2020.

7. WHO. Coronavirus disease 2019 (COVID-19) Situation Report — 72. April 1 2020.

8. WHO — organizational structure. World Health Organization. https://www.who.int/about/who-we-are/structure. Published 2020. Accessed May 25, 2020.

9. 2019 Noval Coronavirus (2019-nCoV) Strategic Preparedness and Response Plan (SPRP) World Health Organization (WHO); Feb 3 2020.

10. WHO. Operational Planning Guidelines to Support Country Preparedness and Response. 2020.

11. COVID-19 Partners Platform. WHO. https://covid-19-response.org/. Published 2020. Accessed.

12. (UNDCO) UDCO. A UN framework for the immediate socio-economic response to COVID-19. United Nations Sustainable Development Group (UNSDG). 2020.

13. ITU-WHO Joint Statement: Unleashing information technology to defeat COVID-19 [press release]. World Health Organization (WHO), Apr 20 2020.

14. EPI-WIN updates. WHO. https://www.who.int/teams/risk-communication/epi-win-updates. Published 2020. Accessed May 31, 2020.

15. WHO UI. Global Communication and Community Engagement Response (RCCE) Strategy to COVID-19 ALNAP May 2 2020.

16. WHO Director-General's opening remarks at the media briefing on 2019 novel coronavirus [press release]. WHO Director-General Speeches: World Health Organization, Feb 6 2020.

17. WHO. Situation Report — 101. World Health Organization (WHO); Apr 30 2020.

18. Director-General speech highlights: OpenWHO [press release]. WHO, Apr 15 2020.
19. Global research and innovation forum to mobilize international action in response to the novel coronavirus (2019-nCoV) emergency. Feb 11–12, 2020; Geneva, Switzerland.
20. WHO. A Coordinated Global Research Roadmap: 2019 Novel Coronavirus. 2020.
21. *Access to COVID-19 Tools (act) Accelerator.* World Health Organization (WHO); Apr 24 2020.
22. World leaders make historic commitments to provide equal access to vaccines for all [press release]. Jun 4 2020.
23. The Access to COVID-19 Tools (ACT) Accelerator. World Health Organization (WHO). Initiatives Web site. https://www.who.int/initiatives/act-accelerator. Published 2020. Accessed July 27, 2020.
24. WHO discontinues hydroxychloroquine and lopinavir/ritonavir treatment arms for COVID-19 [press release]. World Health Organization (WHO), July 4 2020.
25. *Draft landscape of COVID-19 candidate vaccines.* World Health Organization (WHO); Oct 2 2020.
26. Hernández JC. Trump Slammed the W.H.O. Over Coronavirus. He's Not Alone. *New York Times.* Apr 8 2020.
27. Michael R. Pompea SOS. Secretary Michael R. Pompeo With Maria Bartiromo of Mornings with Maria on Fox Business Network. In: Bartiromo M, ed. *Mornings with Maria.* U.S. Department of State 2020.
28. Michael D. Shear DGMJ. Criticized for Pandemic Response, Trump Tries Shifting Blame to the W.H.O. *New York Time.* Apr 14 2020.
29. Donald G. McNeil Jr. AJ. Blaming China for Pandemic, Trump Says U.S. Will Leave the W.H.O. *New York Times.* May 29 2020.
30. Lawrence Gostin SW. Two Legal Experts Explain Why The U.S. Should Not Pull Funding From The WHO Amid COVID-19 Pandemic. In. *Forbes* 2020.
31. Organization WH. "no clear evidence of human-to-human transmission". In: @WHO, ed. *Preliminary investigations conducted by the Chinese authorities have found no clear evidence of human-to-human transmission of the novel #coronavirus (2019-nCoV) identified in #Wuhan, #China*: Twitter; 2020.
32. Ducharme J. The World Health Organization's Maria Van Kerkhove On Balancing Science, Public Relations and Politics. In. *Time* 2020.
33. Novel Coronavirus — China [press release]. World Health Organization (WHO), Jan 12 2020.
34. *Strengthening health security by implementing the International Health Regulations (2005).* World Health Organization (WHO); 2005.

35. WHO Timeline — COVID-19. World Health Organization. https://www.who.int/news-room/detail/27-04-2020-who-timeline---covid-19. Published 2020. Accessed May 25, 2020.

36. *Mission summary: WHO Field Visit to Wuhan, China 20–21 January 2020.* World Health Organization (WHO); Jan 22 2020.

37. Chan JF-W, Yuan S, Kok K-H, *et al.* A familial cluster of pneumonia associated with the 2019 novel coronavirus indicating person-to-person transmission: a study of a family cluster. *The Lancet* 2020;**395**(10223):514–523.

38. Updated WHO recommendations for international traffic in relation to COVID-19 outbreak [press release]. World Health Organization (WHO), Feb 29 2020.

39. Chinazzi M, Davis JT, Ajelli M, *et al.* The effect of travel restrictions on the spread of the 2019 novel coronavirus (COVID-19) outbreak. *Science.* 2020;**368**(6489):395–400.

40. Continued Stringent Implementation & Enforcement of Circuit Breaker Measures [press release]. Apr 14 2020.

41. Wei WE, Li Z, Chiew CJ, Yong SE, Toh MP, Lee VJ. Presymptomatic Transmission of SARS-CoV-2 — Singapore, January 23-March 16, 2020. *MMWR Morb Mortal Wkly Rep.* 2020;**69**(14):411–415.

42. He X, Lau EHY, Wu P, *et al.* Temporal dynamics in viral shedding and transmissibility of COVID-19. *Nat Med.* 2020;**26**(5):672–675.

43. Final update: STAG-IH views on mask use by the general public [press release]. World Health Organization (WHO), May 25 2020.

44. WHO Director-General's opening remarks at the media briefing on COVID-19 — 5 June 2020 [press release]. WHO Director-General, Speeches: WHO, Jun 5 2020.

45. *Report of the WHO-China Joint Mission on Coronavirus Disease 2019 (COVID-19)* World Health Organization; Feb 16–24 2020.

46. Li Q, Guan X, Wu P, *et al.* Early Transmission Dynamics in Wuhan, China, of Novel Coronavirus-Infected Pneumonia. *N Engl J Med.* 2020.

47. One-minute video: How China built Leishenshan Hospital in 10 days. In: YouTube: CGTN; 2020.

48. Kai Kupferschmidt JC. China's aggressive measures have slowed the coronavirus. They may not work in other countries. *Science.* 2020.

49. Claire Che DL, Rachel Chang, Daniela Wei. Overwhelmed Chinese Hospitals Turn Away Patients Without Virus. *Bloomberg.* Feb 21 2020.

50. Coronavirus Pandemic (COVID-19). 2020. https://ourworldindata.org/coronavirus.

51. China to Lift Lockdown Over Virus Epicenter Wuhan on April 8. *Bloomberg*. Mar 24 2020.

52. Claire Che YW. How China Tested 11 Million People for Virus in Just Two Weeks. *Bloomberg*. May 30 2020.

53. A cluster of COVID-19 in Beijing, People's Republic of China [press release]. Jun 13 2020.

54. Holshue ML, DeBolt C, Lindquist S, *et al*. First Case of 2019 Novel Coronavirus in the United States. *N Engl J Med*. 2020;**382**(10):929–936.

55. First Travel-related Case of 2019 Novel Coronavirus Detected in United States [press release]. CDC Newsroom Releases: CDC, Jan 21 2020.

56. From SARS to Coronavirus: Examining the Role of Global Aviation in Containing the Spread of Infectious Disease. In. *Congressional Testimony of the Department of Health and Human Services on COVID-19*. CDC: Senate Commerce, Science, and Transportation Subcommittee on Aviation and Space; 2020.

57. Transcript of Update on 2019 Novel Coronavirus (2019-nCoV) [press release]. CDC Newsroom Releases: CDC, Jan 21 2020.

58. Hillary Leung AG, Sanya Mansoor. A Second Travel-Related Case of Coronavirus Has Been Confirmed in the U.S. Here's What to Know. In. *Time*2020.

59. CDC Advises Travelers to Avoid All Nonessential Travel to China [press release]. CDC, Jan 28 2020.

60. Soucheray S. CDC quarantines 195 passengers; US declares nCoV public health emergency. Center for Infectious Disease Research and Policy. CIDRAP News Web site. https://www.cidrap.umn.edu/news-perspective/2020/01/cdc-quarantines-195-passengers-us-declares-ncov-public-health-emergency. Published 2020. Accessed.

61. Eric Lipton AG, Michael D. Shear, Megan Twohey, Apoorva Mandavilli, Sheri Fink and Mark Walker. "The C.D.C. waited its entire existence for this moment. What went wrong?". *The New York Times*. Jun 3, 2020.

62. Schwellenbach N. *The First 100 Days of the U.S. Government's COVID-19 Response*. POGO; May 6 2020.

63. Transcript for CDC Telebriefing: CDC Update on Novel Coronavirus [press release]. CDC, Feb 12 2020.

64. Shawn Boburg ROHJ, Neena Satija, Amy Goldstein. Inside the coronavirus testing failure: Alarm and dismay among the scientists who sought to help. *The Washington Post*. Apr 3, 2020.

65. Coronavirus Patient and Precautions at UC Davis Medical Center, Robust Infection Control Protocols in Place [press release]. UC Davis, Feb 26 2020.

66. Coronavirus (COVID-19) Update: FDA Issues New Policy to Help Expedite Availability of Diagnostics [press release]. US Food & Drug Administration, Feb 29 2020.

67. Jorden MA RS, et al. Evidence for Limited Early Spread of COVID-19 Within the United States, January–February 2020. *MMWR Morb Mortal Wkly Rep.* **2020**(69):680–684.

68. Ehley B. Trump's team shifts tone from preventing coronavirus to containing it. In: Politico; 2020.

69. 15 Days to Slow the Spread [press release]. Healthcare: The White House, Mar 16 2020.

70. Protecting Healthcare Workers During the COVID-19 Pandemic: A Survey of Infection Preventionists [press release]. Association for Professionals in Infection Control and Epidemiology (APIC), Mar 27 2020.

71. Ranney M. The Demand Data Hub: Powering a Collaborative PPE Supply Chain. In. Medium: ProjectN95; 2020.

72. Gondi S, Beckman AL, Deveau N, et al. Personal protective equipment needs in the USA during the COVID-19 pandemic. *The Lancet.* 2020;**395**(10237): e90–e91.

73. GetUsPPE Announces Publication in The Lancet on Continued Healthcare PPE Shortage in the US [press release]. GetUsPPE.org: GetUsPPE, May 15 2020.

74. Haffajee RL, Mello MM. Thinking Globally, Acting Locally — The U.S. Response to Covid-19. *New England Journal of Medicine.* 2020; **382**(22):e75.

75. WHO Emergencies Press Conference on coronavirus disease outbreak — 13 March 2020 [press release]. World Health Organization, Mar 13 2020.

76. Moss P, Barlow G, Easom N, Lillie P, Samson A. Lessons for managing high-consequence infections from first COVID-19 cases in the UK. *The Lancet.* 2020;**395**(10227).

77. Statement from the 4 UK Chief Medical Officers on novel coronavirus: Update on the UK risk level regarding novel coronavirus [press release]. GOV.UK: Department of Health and Social Care, Jan 30 2020.

78. Spiteri G, Fielding J, Diercke M, et al. First cases of coronavirus disease 2019 (COVID-19) in the WHO European Region, 24 January to 21 February 2020. *Euro Surveill.* 2020;**25**(9):2000178.

79. COVID-19: guidance for staff in the transport sector. Public Health England (PHE). https://web.archive.org/web/20200220133756/https://www.gov.uk/government/publications/covid-19-guidance-for-staff-in-the-transport-sector/covid-19-

guidance-for-staff-in-the-transport-sector. Published 2020. Updated Feb 14. Accessed.

80. REVEALED 38 DAYS when Britain sleepwalked into carnage; Boris Johnson skipped five Cobra meetings on the virus, no protective gear was ordered, and scientists were ignored. Failings in February may have cost lives. *Sunday Times (London, England)*. 2020/04/19/, 2020:10.

81. Health Secretary announces strengthened legal powers to bolster public health protections against coronavirus [press release]. GOV.UK: Department of Health and Social Care, Feb 10 2020.

82. COVID-19: Health Secretary's statement to Parliament: The Secretary of State for Health and Social Care Matt Hancock updated Parliament on the government's response to coronavirus [press release]. GOV.UK: Department of Health and Social Care Feb 26 2020.

83. *Coronavirus: action plan; A guide to what you can expect across the UK.* Department of Health & Social Care; 3 Mar 2020.

84. PM statement at coronavirus press conference: 3 March 2020 [press release]. GOV.UK: Prime Minister's Office Mar 3 2020.

85. Perigo B. Coronavirus Could Hit the U.K. Harder Than Any Other European Country. Here's What Went Wrong. In. *Time*2020.

86. PM statement on coronavirus: 12 March 2020 [press release]. GOV.UK: Prime Minister's Office, Mar 12 2020.

87. PM statement on coronavirus: 18 March 2020 [press release]. GOV.UK: Prime Minister's Office, Mar 18 2020.

88. Hunter DJ. Covid-19 and the Stiff Upper Lip — The Pandemic Response in the United Kingdom. *N Engl J Med*. 2020;**382**(16):e31.

89. PM statement on coronavirus: 16 March 2020 [press release]. GOV.UK: Prime Minister's Office, Mar 16 2020.

90. Yong E. The U.K.'s Coronavirus 'Herd Immunity' Debacle. In. *The Atlantic*2020.

91. Alwan NA, Bhopal R, Burgess RA, *et al.* Evidence informing the UK's COVID-19 public health response must be transparent. *The Lancet.* 2020;**395**(10229):1036–1037.

92. Neil M Ferguson DL, Gemma Nedjati-Gilani, *et al.* Impact of non-pharmaceutical interventions (NPIs) to reduce COVID-19 mortality and healthcare demand. *Imperial College London (16-03-2020)*. 2020.

93. PM statement on coronavirus: 19 March 2020 [press release]. GOV.UK: Prime Minister's Office, Mar 19 2020.

94. Government announces further measures on social distancing [press release]. GOV.UK: Ministry of Housing, Communities & Local Government Mar 20 2020.

95. 22 DAYS How three weeks of dither and delay at No 10 cost thousands of British lives; Scientists, politicians, academics and advisers reveal the inside story of British ministers' desperate battle with the virus in the three weeks before lockdown. *Sunday Times (London, England)*. 2020/05/24/, 2020: 10.

96. Leo Ewbank JT, Helen McKenna, Siva Anandaciva. NHS hospital bed numbers: past, present, future. *The King's Fund*. 2020.

97. McCarthy N. The Countries With The Most Critical Care Beds Per Capita. https://www.statista.com/chart/21105/number-of-critical-care-beds-per-100000-inhabitants/. Published 2020. Updated Mar 12. Accessed.

98. Paul Nuki BG. Exercise Cygnus uncovered: the pandemic warnings buried by the government *The Telegraph*. Mar 28, 2020.

99. Health and Social Care Secretary's statement on coronavirus (COVID-19): 3 April 2020 [press release]. GOV.UK: Department of Health and Social Care Apr 3 2020.

100. Charlie Haynes JC. Coronavirus: Doctors 'told not to discuss PPE shortages'. *BBC*. May 15, 2020.

101. Shepherd A. Covid-19: Frontline doctors continue PPE fight. *BMJ*. 2020; **369**:m2188.

102. Andrew Gregory NH, Sian Griffiths. Coronavirus crisis: doctors take legal action to force inquiry into PPE shortage. *The Sunday Times*. May 10, 2020.

103. Coronavirus (COVID-19) roundup: Deaths involving COVID-19. Office of National Statistics. https://www.ons.gov.uk/peoplepopulationandcommunity/healthandsocialcare/conditionsanddiseases/articles/coronaviruscovid19roundup/2020-03-26#coviddeaths. Published 2020. Accessed.

104. Oliver Pybus AR, Louis du Plessis, Alexander E Zarebski, Moritz UG Kraemer, Jayna Raghwani, Bernardo Gutiérrez, Verity Hill, John McCrone, Rachel, Colquhoun, Ben Jackson, Áine O'Toole, Jordan Ashworth, on behalf of the COG-UK consortium. Preliminary analysis of SARS-CoV-2 importation & establishment of UK transmission lineages. In: COG-UK consortium; 2020.

105. Phoebe Dunn LA, Genevieve Cameron, Hugh Alderwick. COVID-19 policy tracker. The Health Foundation. https://www.health.org.uk/news-and-comment/charts-and-infographics/covid-19-policy-tracker. Published 2020. Updated Jun 10. Accessed Jun 10.

106. Thomas Hale NA, Rafael Goldszmidt, Beatriz Kira, Anna Petherick, Toby Phillips, Samuel Webster, Emily Cameron-Blake, Laura Hallas, Saptarshi Majumdar, and Helen Tatlow. A global panel database of pandemic policies (Oxford COVID-19 Government Response Tracker. *Nature Human Behaviour*. 2020;2020(Aug 30).

107. Tegnell A. Webinar 26: Case Study in COVID-19 Responses: Lessons Learned from Sweden with Dr. Anders Tegnell. In: Barnathan J, ed: International Center for Journalists (ICFJ); 2020.

108. Decisions and guidelines in the Ministry of Health and Social Affairs' policy areas to limit the spread of the COVID-19 virus [press release]. Government Offices of Sweden: Ministry of Health and Social Affairs, Apr 9 2020.

109. Tegnell A. 'Closing borders is ridiculous': the epidemiologist behind Sweden's controversial coronavirus strategy. In: Paterlini M, ed. News Q&A. Vol 580: Nature; 2020.

110. Apple Mobility Trends. Apple; 2020. https://www.apple.com/covid19/mobility. Accessed Jun 2.

111. Strategy in response to the COVID-19 pandemic [press release]. Government Offices of Swedent: Prime Minister's Office, Apr 6 2020.

112. Public Health Agency: Low proportion of antibodies among elderly. Public Health Agency. https://www.krisinformation.se/en/news/2020/may/antibodies-study. Published 2020. Accessed.

113. Milne R. Sweden unlikely to feel economic benefit of no-lockdown approach. Financial Times. May 10, 2020.

114. Positive Covid tests in no-lockdown Sweden hit lowest rate since pandemic began. Today Online. Sep 9, 2020.

115. Baker M, Kvalsvig A, Verrall AJ, Telfar-Barnard L, Wilson N. New Zealand's elimination strategy for the COVID-19 pandemic and what is required to make it work. N Z Med J. 2020;**133**(1512):10–14.

116. Coronavirus: New Zealand bans travellers from China to 'protect New Zealanders' from deadly virus. The New Zealand Herald. Feb 2, 2020.

117. Single case of COVID-19 confirmed in New Zealand [press release]. Ministry of Health, Feb 28 2020.

118. Immigration update on temporary border closure [press release]. Unite against COVID-19: New Zealand Government, Mar 19 2020.

119. Managed isolation of new arrivals to New Zealand [press release]. Unite against COVID-19: New Zealand Government, Apr 9 2020.

120. Prime Minister Jacinda Ardern — statement to the nation (21/03/20) [press release]. Unite against COVID-19: New Zealand Government, Mar 21 2020.

121. Update from Prime Minister Jacinda Ardern (23/03/20) [press release]. Unite against COVID-19: New Zealand Government, Mar 23 2020.

122. State of National Emergency declared to fight COVID-19 [press release]. Unite against COVID-19: New Zealand Government, Mar 25 2020.

123. Alert Level 4. New Zealand Government. COVID-19 Alert System Web site. https://covid19.govt.nz/alert-system/alert-level-4/. Published 2020. Updated May 14. Accessed May 31, 2020.

124. COVID-19 — current cases. Ministry of Health, New Zealand. https://www.health.govt.nz/our-work/diseases-and-conditions/covid-19-novel-coronavirus/covid-19-current-situation/covid-19-current-cases. Published 2020. Accessed May 31, 2020.

125. Gunia A. Why New Zealand's Coronavirus Elimination Strategy Is Unlikely to Work in Most Other Places. In. *Time*2020.

126. Duncan G. What is New Zealand's 'elimination strategy' and how has it united the country? *World Economic Forum, The Conversation*. 2020.

127. Cousins S. New Zealand eliminates COVID-19. *The Lancet*. 2020;**395**(10235).

128. Daily COVID-19 media conference — 27 April [press release]. Unite against COVID-19: New Zealand Government, Apr 27 2020.

129. New Zealand will be at Alert Level 2 from Thursday 14 May [press release]. Unite against COVID-19: New Zealand Government, May 11 2020.

130. Upcoming changes to gathering numbers [press release]. Unite against COVID-19: New Zealand Government, May 25 2020.

131. Transcript of the 11 August media conference [press release]. Aug 11 2020.

132. 4 new cases of COVID-19 [press release]. Sep 7 2020.

133. Phan LT, Nguyen TV, Luong QC, et al. Importation and Human-to-Human Transmission of a Novel Coronavirus in Vietnam. *New England Journal of Medicine*. 2020;**382**(9):872–874.

134. Markovitz G. To test or not to test? Two experts explain COVID-19 testing. *World Economic Forum*. 2020.

135. Guy Thwaites MR, Marc Choisy, Rogier van Doorn, Duong Huy Luong, Dang Quang Tan, Tran Dai Quang, Phung Cong Dinh, Ngu Duy Nghia, Tran Anh Tu, La Ngoc Quang, Nguyen Cong Khanh, Dang Duc Anh, Tran Nhu Duong, Sang Minh Le, Thai Pham Quang. *Emerging COVID-19 success story: Vietnam's commitment to containment*. Our World in Data June 30 2020.

136. GardaWorld. *Vietnam: Son Loi (Vinh Phuc province) placed under quarantine due to coronavirus February 13 /update 7*. GardaWorld News Alerts Feb 14 2020.

137. Khanh Vu PN, James Pearson. After aggressive mass testing, Vietnam says it contains coronavirus outbreak. *Reuters*. Apr 30, 2020.

138. Nguyen Dieu Tu Uyen XQN, Mai Ngoc Chau. Vietnam's No Virus Death Record Ends With Hospital Outbreak. *Bloomberg*. Aug 8, 2020.

139. Hui Sin Teo SB, Caryn Bredenkamp, Jewelwayne Salcedo Cain. *The Future of Health Financing in Vietnam: Ensuring Sufficiency, Efficiency, and Sustainability (English)*. Washington, D.C.: World Bank Group; June 2019.

140. Mortality rate, infant (per 1,000 live births) — Vietnam [data set]. World Bank Data. Washington, DC: World Bank; 2020. https://data.worldbank.org/indicator/SP.DYN.IMRT.IN?locations=VN. Accessed Aug 31, 2020.

141. (WHO) WHO. *Joint External Evaluation of IHR Core Capacities of Viet Nam*. Geneva: WHO;2017.

142. CDC. Vietnam: Connecting for Stronger Emergency Response. CDC and the Global Health Security Agenda Web site. https://www.cdc.gov/globalhealth/security/stories/vietnam_emergency_response.html. Published 2016. Updated May 17, 2016. Accessed Aug 31, 2020.

143. Field epidemiology training programme in Viet Nam. Health Topics Web site. https://www.who.int/vietnam/health-topics/field-epidemiology-training-program-(fetp). Published 2020. Accessed Aug 31, 2020.

144. Balajee SA, Pasi O, Etoundi AG, et al. Sustainable Model for Public Health Emergency Operations Centers for Global Settings. *Emerging Infectious Disease journal*. 2017;**23**(13).

145. CDC. Vietnam Update: Community-Based Surveillance Yields Results. Global Health Protection and Security Web site. https://www.cdc.gov/globalhealth/healthprotection/fieldupdates/summer-2017/vietnam-community-surveillance.html. Published 2019. Accessed Aug 31, 2020.

146. Cobelens FG, Harris VC. Untangling SARS-CoV-2 epidemic control — lessons from Vietnam. *Clin Infect Dis*. 2020.

147. O'Kane C. Catchy PSA about coronavirus turns into viral TikTok challenge about washing your hands. *CBS News*. Mar 4, 2020.

148. COVID-19: government handling and confidence in health authorities. 2020. https://today.yougov.com/topics/international/articles-reports/2020/03/17/perception-government-handling-covid-19. Accessed Aug 31, 2020.

149. Staff AB. Southeast Asia's GDP growth to contract by 4.2% in 2020; Vietnam recovery prospects brightest: ICAEW. *The Business Times*. Sep 7, 2020.

150. Joanna Slater NM. India surpasses Brazil to take second spot in total coronavirus cases. *The Washington Post*. Sep 7, 2020; Asia & Pacific.

151. Jeffrey Gettleman SY. India's Covid Outbreak Is Now the World's Fastest-Growing. *The New York Times*. Aug 28, 2020.

152. WHO. *India Situation Report — 2*.Feb 6 2020.

153. Ipchita Bharali PK, Sakthivel Selvaraj. *How well is India responding to COVID-19?*: Brookings; July 2 2020.

154. Coronavirus: India cancels valid visas to Chinese, foreigners who visited China in last two weeks. *The Indian Express.* Feb 4, 2020.

155. WHO. *India Situation Report — 6.*Mar 28 2020.

156. Ghosh J. A critique of the Indian government's response to the COVID-19 pandemic. *Journal of Industrial and Business Economics.* 2020;**47**(3):519–530.

157. WHO. *India Situation Report — 16.*May 17 2020.

158. WHO. *India Situation Report — 18.*May 31 2020.

159. Iyer M. One in four Indians may have Covid antibodies, show tests. *Times of India.* Aug 19, 2020.

160. Crump A. Japan's coronavirus response is flawed — but it works. *Nikkei Asian Review.* May 14, 2020.

161. Murakami H. Japan's Response to Covid-19 is Prudent. *Center for Strategic & International Studies (CSIS).* 2020;**3**(4).

162. Lancet T. COVID-19 in Brazil: "So what?". *Lancet.* 2020;**395**(10235):1461.

163. Coronavirus: Hard-hit Brazil removes data amid rising death toll. *BBC News.* Jun 7, 2020.

164. Gram Slattery PF. Bolsonaro Calls WHO 'Political,' Threatens Brazil Exit. *New York Times.* Jun 6, 2020.

165. KA Moore ML, JM Barry, MT Osterholm *Part 1: The Future of the COVID-19 Pandemic: Lessons Learned from Pandemic Influenza.* Center for Infectious Disease Research and Policy (CIDRAP); April 30, 2020.

166. Ho R. Commentary: China's COVID-19 successes — credible at home, not so much abroad. *Channel News Asia.* Jul 4, 2021.

167. Boeing P, Wang Y. Decoding China's COVID-19 'virus exceptionalism': Community-based digital contact tracing in Wuhan. *R&D Management.* n/a(n/a).

168. Firestone MJ, Wienkes H, Garfin J, *et al.* COVID-19 Outbreak Associated with a 10-Day Motorcycle Rally in a Neighboring State — Minnesota, August-September 2020. *MMWR Morb Mortal Wkly Rep.* 2020;**69**(47):1771–1776.

169. Bernheim BDab, Nina and Freitas-Groff, Zach and Otero, Sebastián. *The Effects of Large Group Meetings on the Spread of COVID-19: The Case of Trump Rallies (October 30, 2020).* SSRN Oct 30, 2020.

170. Lewis T. How the U.S. Pandemic Response Went Wrong—and What Went Right—during a Year of COVID. In. *Scientific American*2021.

171. Covid-19: UK reports a record 55,892 daily cases. *BBC.* Dec 31, 2020.

172. Kirby T. New variant of SARS-CoV-2 in UK causes surge of COVID-19. *Lancet Respir Med.* 2021;**9**(2):e20–e21.

173. Covid: New lockdowns for England and Scotland ahead of 'hardest weeks'. *BBC*. Jan. 2021.

174. Triggle N. Hospital pressure forces PM's hand. *BBC*. Jan 5, 2021.

175. WHO warns of 'two-track pandemic' as cases decline but vaccine inequity persists [press release]. UN News, Jun 7 2021.

176. Claeson M, Hanson S. The Swedish COVID-19 strategy revisited. *The Lancet*. 2021;**397**(10285):1619.

177. Willoughby E. *An ideal public health model? Vietnam's state-led, preventative, low-cost response to COVID-19*. Brookings; Jun 29 2021.

178. Kugelman M. How India Became Pandemic Ground Zero. In. *Foreign Policy*. South Asia Brief2021.

179. Raut A, Huy NT. Rising incidence of mucormycosis in patients with COVID-19: another challenge for India amidst the second wave? *The Lancet Respiratory Medicine*.

180. Repurposed Antiviral Drugs for Covid-19 — Interim WHO Solidarity Trial Results. *New England Journal of Medicine*. 2020;**384**(6):497–511.

181. COVAX https://www.gavi.org/covax-facility. Published 2021. Accessed Jul 26, 2021.

182. WHO chief says 'don't politicize' COVID-19 after Trump criticism. *Reuters*. Apr 9, 2020.

183. Flaxman S, Mishra S, Gandy A, *et al.* Estimating the effects of non-pharmaceutical interventions on COVID-19 in Europe. *Nature*. 2020;**584**(7820):257–261.

184. Leacock M. No Single Player Can Win This Board Game. It's Called Pandemic. *New York Times*. March 25, 2020;Opinion.

185. Wallace S. Disaster looms for indigenous Amazon tribes as COVID-19 cases multiply. In. *National Geographic*2020.

186. Times TNY. India Coronavirus Map and Case Count. In:2020.

187. WHO, China leaders discuss next steps in battle against coronavirus outbreak [press release]. World Health Organization (WHO), Jan 28 2020.

188. UN releases US$15 million to help vulnerable countries battle the spread of the coronavirus [press release]. Mar 1 2020.

189. WHO Director-General calls on G20 to Fight, Unite, and Ignite against COVID-19 [press release]. World Health Organization (WHO), Mar 26 2020.

190. WHO releases guidelines to help countries maintain essential health services during the COVID-19 pandemic [press release]. World Health Organization (WHO), Mar 30 2020.

191. WHO and UNICEF to partner on pandemic response through COVID-19 Solidarity Response Fund [press release]. World Health Organization (WHO), Apr 3 2020.

192. 'One World: Together At Home' Raised Almost $128 Million in Response to the COVID-19 Crisis [press release]. Global Citizen, Apr 19 2020.

193. WHO and Global Citizen announce: 'One World: Together at home' Global Special to support healthcare workers in the fight against the COVID-19 pandemic [press release]. World Health Organization (WHO), Apr 6 2020.

194. Statement on the third meeting of the International Health Regulations (2005) Emergency Committee regarding the outbreak of coronavirus disease (COVID-19) [press release]. World Health Organization (WHO), May 1 2020.

195. ECOSOC Informal Briefing on 'Joining Forces: Effective Policy Solutions for Covid-19 Response' [press release]. World Health Organization (WHO), May 11 2020.

196. *Rational use of personal protective equipment for coronavirus disease (COVID-19) and considerations during severe shortages.* World Health Organization; Feb 27 2020.

197. Shortage of personal protective equipment endangering health workers worldwide [press release]. World Health Organization (WHO), Mar 3 2020.

198. Pandemic Supply Chain Network (PSCN). World Economic Forum. https://www.weforum.org/covid-action-platform/projects/pandemic-supply-chain-network-pscn. Published 2020. Accessed May 25, 2020.

199. WHO COVID-19 Essential Supplies Forecasting Tool (ESFT). WHO. Coronavirus disease (COVID-19) technical guidance: Essential resource planning Web site. https://www.who.int/emergencies/diseases/novel-coronavirus-2019/technical-guidance/covid-19-critical-items. Updated April 29, 2020. Accessed May 12, 2020.

200. Gavi Board calls for global access to COVID-19 vaccines [press release]. Jun 26 2020.

201. "Emerging respiratory viruses, including nCoV: methods for detection, prevention, response and control" now available [press release]. WHO, Jan 25 2020.

202. Pass the message: Five steps to kicking out coronavirus [press release]. World Health Organization Mar 23 2020.

203. Launch of the WHO Academy and the WHO Info mobile applications [press release]. World Health Organization (WHO), May 13 2020.

204. WHO to accelerate research and innovation for new coronavirus [press release]. World Health Organization (WHO), Feb 6 2020.

205. Global research on coronavirus disease (COVID-19). World Health Organization. https://www.who.int/emergencies/diseases/novel-coronavirus-2019/global-research-on-novel-coronavirus-2019-ncov. Published 2020. Accessed May 12, 2020.

206. Global leaders unite to ensure everyone everywhere can access new vaccines, tests and treatments for COVID-19 [press release]. World Health Organization (WHO), Apr 24 2020.

207. "Solidarity" clinical trial for COVID-19 treatments WHO. https://www.who.int/emergencies/diseases/novel-coronavirus-2019/global-research-on-novel-coronavirus-2019-ncov/solidarity-clinical-trial-for-covid-19-treatments. Published 2020. Accessed Jun 13, 2020.

Epidemiology of COVID-19

Calvin J Chiew, Zongbin Li and Vernon J Lee

Our understanding of the virus and disease continues to evolve as new scientific evidence emerges. The information presented in this chapter represents the state of knowledge as of writing.

Overview of the Outbreak

Global

At the end of 2019, a cluster of pneumonia cases suspected to be caused by a new virus was reported in Wuhan, a city in the Hubei Province of China. In February 2020, the World Health Organization (WHO) designated the disease COVID-19. The virus was designated as severe acute respiratory syndrome coronavirus 2 (SARS-CoV-2); previously, it was referred to as 2019-nCoV.

Since the first reports of COVID-19 at the end of 2019, the infection has spread rapidly to more than 20 million confirmed cases worldwide by mid-August 2020, affecting all continents except Antarctica. This prompted the WHO to declare a public health emergency of international concern on 30 January 2020 and characterise it as a pandemic on 11 March 2020.

The reported case counts likely underestimate the true burden of COVID-19, as only a fraction of acute infections is diagnosed by PCR tests. Seroprevalence surveys in the United States (US) and Europe suggest that the true rate of infection exceeds the incidence of reported cases by approximately 10-fold (McIntosh, 2020).

Singapore

Singapore reported its first case of COVID-19 on 23 January 2020, in a traveller from Wuhan. Three overlapping waves of infection can be described in the local outbreak. The first wave in January–February 2020 consisted of visitors from China, with limited local transmission around them. This was followed by a second wave of imported cases in March 2020 who were mainly Singapore residents returning from other parts of the world as the pandemic epicentre shifted from China to Europe, then the US and beyond. This resulted in greater community transmission and the formation of multiple local clusters, which were contained by the "Circuit Breaker" (CB) community public health measures. The third wave began in April 2020 due to large clusters among migrant workers residing in dormitories; it began to subside in July/August 2020 as a result of specific actions in the dormitories.

Over 55,000 cases have been reported in Singapore by mid-August 2020, the majority (>95%) of whom are dormitory residents. Due to the migrant worker population being disproportionately affected, most of the cases are males aged 20–40 years. About 700 cases were imported while the rest were locally acquired.

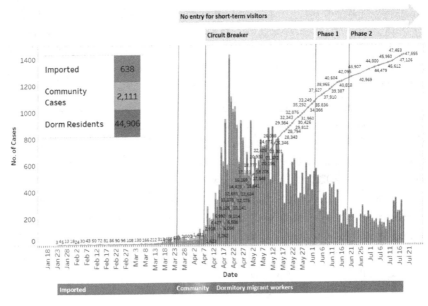

Figure 1.   Epidemic curve of COVID-19 infections in Singapore, 2020.

Virus/disease Characteristics

Mode of transmission

Transmission of SARS-CoV-2 occurs primarily between people through close contact, either through infected secretions such as saliva and respiratory secretions or through respiratory droplets, expelled when an infected person coughs, sneezes, talks or sings (World Health Organization, 2020). Respiratory droplets are >5–10 µm in diameter and usually land within 1–2 metres of the infected person; they may reach the eyes, nose or mouth of a susceptible person, resulting in infection.

Respiratory secretions or droplets can also contaminate surfaces and objects, creating fomites. Fomite transmission is thought to be likely, due to consistent evidence showing environmental contamination and survival of the virus on certain surfaces, although no specific reports have directly demonstrated it. In a Singapore study, viral RNA was detected on nearly all surfaces tested (handles, light switches, bed and handrails, interior doors and windows, toilet bowl, and sink basin) in the isolation room of a COVID-19 patient prior to routine cleaning (Ong et al., 2020).

Airborne transmission of the virus can occur during medical procedures that generate aerosols (droplet nuclei), which are respiratory droplets <5 µm in diameter and can remain suspended in the air over long distances and time. An air sampling study in Singapore detected positive particles of sizes 1–4 µm and >4 µm in two isolation rooms (Chia et al., 2020). Outbreak reports related to indoor crowded spaces have suggested the possibility of aerosol transmission in the community as well since coughing, sneezing and singing could potentially generate aerosols (Morawska and Milton, 2020). However, the role and extent of airborne transmission outside of healthcare settings, in particular, closed settings with poor ventilation, is still controversial and under further study.

Viral RNA has also been detected in non-respiratory samples, including stool, urine, blood, semen and tears (McIntosh, 2020; World Health Organization, 2020; Centers for Disease Control and Prevention, 2020). In addition, the infection has been described in animals both in natural and experimental settings. However, there have been no published cases of fecal-oral, bloodborne, sexual, mother-to-child and animal-to-human transmission thus far.

Incubation period

The median incubation period (time from infection to symptom onset) for COVID-19 is 4–5 days but can be as long as 14 days (Centers for Disease Control and Prevention, 2020),[6] similar to SARS and MERS. One study reported that 97.5% of COVID-19 patients who developed symptoms did so within 11.5 days of infection (Lauer et al., 2020).

In a study of 77 well-characterised infector-infectee pairs from Hong Kong, the mean serial interval (the period between symptom onset of a primary case to symptom onset of its secondary case) of COVID-19 was 5.8 days (He et al., 2020).

In line with international findings, cases in Singapore have a mean incubation period of five days [unpublished MOH data]. A study on three clusters in Singapore found the serial interval between transmission pairs ranged between 3–8 days (Pung et al., 2020).

Severity of illness, subclinical/asymptomatic rate

In a large cohort of >44,000 confirmed cases from China, 81% had mild to moderate disease (mild symptoms up to mild pneumonia), 14% had severe disease (dyspnea, hypoxia, or >50% lung involvement on imaging), and 5% had critical disease (respiratory failure, shock, or multiorgan system dysfunction) (Chinese Chinese Center for Disease Control and Prevention, 2020).

Infection has been documented in asymptomatic and pre-asymptomatic individuals. Since persons without symptoms are not routinely tested, estimating the prevalence of asymptomatic infection in the population is difficult. A wide range of estimates, from 4% to 80%, has been suggested in the literature. A meta-analysis obtained a pooled estimate of 15% for the proportion of truly asymptomatic cases (Byambasuren et al., 2020). A study from China, which clearly defined asymptomatic infections with appropriate follow-up, suggested that the asymptomatic rate was 23% (Wang et al., 2020). Studies also show that children are more likely to be asymptomatic and to have milder illnesses compared to adults (Centers for Disease Control and Prevention, 2020; Ng et al., 2020).

In Singapore, a large proportion (>70%) of the community cases were asymptomatic, mostly detected via active surveillance or case finding. In a cohort of 80 patients, 21% required oxygen supplementation, 14% required

HD/ICU care, and 10% required mechanical ventilation [unpublished NCID data]. A case report highlighted a 6-month-old infant who tested PCR positive up to day 16 of admission despite being largely asymptomatic (Kam *et al.*, 2020).

Mortality rate, high-risk groups

Globally, more than 750,000 deaths caused by COVID-19 have been reported by mid-August 2020. The case fatality rate (number of deaths over the number of confirmed cases) varies across countries due to numerous factors including the availability of testing and ICU care. In the cohort of >44,000 confirmed cases in China, the overall case fatality rate was 2.3% (Chinese Center for Disease Control and Prevention, 2020). Within a captive cohort onboard the Diamond Princess cruise ship, a case fatality rate of 1% was observed (Rajgor *et al.*, 2020). This makes COVID-19 more lethal than H1N1 (CFR of about 0.1%) but less than SARS (CRF of about 10%).

Estimating the infection fatality rate (number of deaths over the number of actual infections) requires knowing the mildly symptomatic and asymptomatic rate, which is still uncertain due to the lack of testing of these cases. A meta-analysis of 25 studies obtained an estimated infection fatality rate of 0.64% (Meyerowitz-Katz and Merone, 2020). Serological studies could indicate the true infection rate and burden of disease.

Persons above the age of 65 are at significant risk of severe disease and death from COVID-19, with those aged 50 and above also at higher risk compared to younger persons. The presence of concurrent medical conditions is also associated with increased disease severity and mortality. These include cardiovascular disease, lung disease, chronic kidney disease undergoing dialysis, liver disease, stroke, cancer, immunosuppression, diabetes, hypertension and severe obesity (BMI >40) (Centers for Disease Control and Prevention, 2020).

In Singapore, the case fatality rate has been kept relatively low (<0.1%). Most of the deaths occurred in persons aged 60 and above with chronic comorbidities. Based on an analysis of 2,472 local patients, the proportion of patients requiring oxygen supplementation and ICU care increases with age, with sharp rises at the thresholds of ages 50 and 60 [unpublished NCID data].

Immunity period, reinfection

Infection appears to induce IgM and IgG antibodies generally within two weeks of symptom onset (European Centre for Disease Prevention and Control, 2020), although it is unknown whether all infected individuals mount an immune response, what concentration of antibodies is needed to confer protection, and how long any protective effect will last. Antibodies in other coronaviruses have been shown to wane over time leading to homologous re-infections (Edridge et al., 2020). However, SARS-CoV-2-specific CD4 and CD8 T cell responses have been identified in recovered COVID-19 patients, suggesting the potential for a durable T cell mediated immunity (McIntosh, 2020).

In Singapore, a longitudinal cohort showed that 4% of patients did not seroconvert, and 6% had levels of neutralising antibodies dropping below a 20% cut-off after 90 days [unpublished NCID/PROTECT data]. The magnitude of antibody response appears to correlate with disease severity. A local study found that SARS-recovered patients still possessed long-lasting memory T cells reactive to SARS-NP (nucleocapsid protein) 17 years after the 2003 outbreak (Le Bert et al., 2020).

Four cases of COVID-19 reinfections confirmed by viral genomic sequencing have been reported globally up to October 2020, with interval periods from 48 to 142 days (Iwasaki, 2020). It is still unclear how frequent and severe reinfections are and whether they occur because of inadequate immune response after the first infection. In a report from the Korea Centers for Disease Control and Prevention, the infectious virus could not be cultured on any of the 108 recovered patients who tested PCR positive after being cleared from isolation (Korea Centers for Disease Control and Prevention, 2020). None of their 790 contacts traced to exposure during the period of the repeat positive test developed an infection. In Singapore, recovered cases who test PCR positive again after 90 days have been systematically sent to NCID for evaluation, and no reinfections were confirmed as of October 2020.

Transmission Dynamics

R_0, attack rate

A systematic review of published estimates of the reproductive number (R_0) for COVID-19 found it to be between 2 to 3 (Liu et al., 2020), which is similar in magnitude to SARS (R_0 2–5) and seasonal influenza (R_0 1–2), and lower than airborne viruses such as measles (R_0 12–18) and chickenpox (R_0 10–12).

The secondary attack rate among all close contacts is approximately 0.45% to 0.7% (BMJ Best Practice, 2020). It is higher among household members and ranges from 4.6% to 30%, and lower in children compared to adults (Yung et al., 2020). A large seroprevalence survey from Spain highlighted the greater risk of transmission with having an infected household member, as compared to a co-worker, non-household family member or friend (Pollán et al., 2020).

Modelling of the effective reproduction number (Rt) in Singapore found that it largely remained below 1, except for outbreaks in migrant worker dormitories in April–May [unpublished MOH data]. Seroepidemiological studies showed low seroprevalence among the general population, close contacts of confirmed cases and healthcare workers in Singapore (National Centre for Infectious Diseases, 2020). The overall attack rate was <1% among the general population and 5% among household contacts, while none in a cohort of over 1,000 healthcare workers tested seropositive [unpublished NCID data]. Household contacts were more likely to be infected than workplace, social or transport-related contacts [unpublished MOH data]. Consistent with international findings, the local risk of infection in the household setting increases with age [unpublished MOH data].

Period/duration of infectiousness, viral shedding

SARS-CoV-2 viral RNA can be detected in cases 1–3 days before their symptom onset, with the highest viral loads (as measured by PCR) observed around the day of symptom onset, followed by a gradual decline over time (World Health Organization, 2020; He et al., 2020; Wölfel et al., 2020). As such, COVID-19 patients are more infectious in the early course of illness, in contrast to SARS, where viral loads peaked 6–11 days after symptom onset (Cheng et al., 2004).

While viral shedding declines with the resolution of symptoms, it may continue for days to weeks (Centers for Disease Control and Prevention, 2020; Young et al., 2020); it appears to be longer in symptomatic cases, more severe diseases and immunocompromised patients (McIntosh, 2020; World Health Organization, 2020). The duration of viral shedding is longer in stool samples than in respiratory and serum samples (Zheng et al., 2020).

However, prolonged viral RNA shedding after symptom resolution is not associated with prolonged infectiousness. A small study from Germany found that the virus could not be cultured from respiratory samples after day 8 of symptom onset (Wölfel et al., 2020). This together with other similar evidence showing the rarity of a viable virus in respiratory samples nine days after symptom onset allowed the WHO to recommend de-isolating patients based on time after symptom onset (or positive test if asymptomatic), rather than on repeated negative PCR results, in May 2020 (World Health Organization, 2020a).

An analysis of 766 patients in Singapore indicated that by day 15 of illness, 30% of COVID-19 patients are PCR-negative by the nasopharyngeal swab. This rises to 68% by day 21, 88% by day 28 and 95% by day 33 (National Centre for Infectious Diseases and Chapter of Infectious Disease Physicians, 2020). A surrogate marker of viral load with PCR is the cycle threshold (Ct) value. A low Ct value indicates a high viral load and vice versa. In a local multicentre cohort of 73 COVID-19 patients, no viable virus (based on being able to culture the virus) was found when the Ct value was 30 or higher. In addition, the virus could not be isolated or cultured after day 11 of illness (National Centre for Infectious Diseases and Chapter of Infectious Disease Physicians, 2020). These data corroborate with international findings that while viral RNA detection may persist in some patients, it represents a non-viable virus and such patients are non-infectious.

Asymptomatic/re-symptomatic transmission

Multiple studies have documented SARS-CoV-2 transmission during the pre-symptomatic incubation period, which is supported by viral shedding data (see previous section) (World Health Organization, 2020; CDC, 2020). A viable virus has also been isolated from an asymptomatic case (World Health Organization, 2020a).

However, the extent to which asymptomatic or pre-symptomatic transmission occurs and how much it contributes to the pandemic remains unknown. A study in Singapore identified 6.4% of patients among seven clusters of cases in which pre-symptomatic transmission was likely to have occurred 1–3 days before symptom onset (Wei et al., 2020).

It is believed that individuals without symptoms are less likely to transmit the virus than symptomatic persons. Four studies from Brunei, China, Taiwan and the Republic of Korea found that between 0% and 2.2% of asymptomatic cases infected someone else, compared to 0.8%–15.4% of symptomatic cases (World Health Organization, 2020).

Risk factors for transmission

The risk of transmission increases with closeness and duration of contact with infected individuals and appears highest with prolonged close contact in indoor settings. Most secondary infections globally have been described in household settings, in congregate settings where individuals are in close quarters (such as cruise ships, homeless shelters, detention facilities and meat processing facilities), and in healthcare settings where personal protective equipment was inadequate or not used (including hospitals and long-term care facilities) (McIntosh, 2020).

In an analysis of 75,465 COVID-19 cases in China, 78–85% of clusters occurred within household settings (World Health Organization, 2020b). Outside of the household setting, clusters of cases have originated from workplaces, social gatherings, parties and weddings, gyms and fitness classes, and places of worship where close personal contact can occur (BMJ Best Practice, 2020). An outbreak among a choir group with a high attack rate raised the possibility of transmission risk through singing in close proximity (Hamner et al., 2020).

The clusters in Singapore were mainly in households and dormitories, although there were also interesting clusters in workplaces, social settings, religious gatherings and nursing homes. A study on three local clusters (at a complementary health products shop, a company conference, and a church) found direct or prolonged close contact among affected individuals, as well as potential indirect transmission via fomites and shared food (Pung et al., 2020). Several non-household clusters were seeded by individuals who continued to work or partake in social activities despite being ill.

Clusters at a private dinner function with singing performances and at several churches with congregational singing suggest that singing is a high-risk activity. The volume of respiratory droplets emitted during singing is six times compared to normal talking and equivalent to that produced by coughing (Asadi *et al.*, 2019). The large clusters in migrant worker dormitories exemplify the vulnerability of close living environments for rapid transmission. Network analysis found construction worksites to be hubs of transmission among migrant workers residing in different dormitories.

Consistent with international findings that young children are less affected than adults, schools did not emerge as high-risk settings. In two Singapore pre-school outbreaks mostly involving adult staff, all of the students identified as close contacts and tested turned out negative for COVID-19 [unpublished MOH data].

Implications for Public Health Response

Case detection

The first step to the containment of the COVID-19 outbreak requires robust case detection for rapid isolation of cases and contact tracing. Singapore used a combination of detecting cases among symptomatic patients who present at clinics, active case findings, and various surveillance systems to detect COVID-19 cases (Table 1).

Active case finding and active surveillance detected the majority of confirmed cases, accounting for about 85% of case detection as a result of testing among high-risk individuals. Case definition accounted for a further 15%, with only several cases detected through other surveillance systems.

Table 1. Case detection methods used In Singapore.

Patients Who Present At Clinics	Active Case Finding	Active Surveillance	Other Surveillance Systems
• Suspect case definition • Swab-and-send-home (SASH) • Doctor's discretion	• Ring-fencing around confirmed cases • Entry/exit screening for persons under quarantine (PUQs) and persons on Stay-Home Notice (SHN) • Regional screening around clusters	• Community screening and routine regular testing of target groups (e.g., foreign workers in dormitories, nursing homes, pre-schools, and frontline staff)	• Influenza-like-illness (ILI)/acute respiratory illness (ARI) • Severe illness and death from possibly infectious causes (SIDPIC)

Patients who present at clinics

The suspect case definition was first developed on 2 January 2020, days after China reported a cluster of pneumonia cases in Wuhan, Hubei Province. All medical practitioners and healthcare institutions were updated of the suspect case definition, which included a combination of clinical signs and symptoms and epidemiological history (e.g., travel to high-risk areas or contact history). As the outbreak progressed and with growing knowledge of the disease, the suspect case definition was regularly updated. For example, as more countries reported exponential increases of confirmed cases, the list of countries considered high-risk gradually expanded to include all countries. To account for the local situation involving foreign workers in dormitories, any individual who stayed in a foreign worker dormitory was also considered high-risk.

An addition to the suspect case definition was the swab-and-send-home (SASH) criteria. The enhanced criteria sought to expand the availability of testing to symptomatic individuals with an acute respiratory infection (ARI) who do not fulfill the suspect case definition. As Singapore's testing capacity was scaled-up, the criteria were expanded on 1 July 2020 from testing those who stay in congregated settings to eventually include any individual aged 13 years and above with ARI.

To allow for flexibility, doctors could also perform testing for cases at their own discretion if the patient was deemed to have a suggestive clinical or epidemiological history.

Active case finding

Due to the possibility of transmission from confirmed cases to their contacts, active case finding was performed around confirmed cases. With increasing evidence of pre-symptomatic transmission based on local and global data, contact tracing and isolation of close contacts was extended from the date of symptom onset to two days prior to symptom onset. All contacts of confirmed cases were identified and classified based on proximity and duration of contact. To aid in activity mapping for contact tracing, digital solutions were developed. SafeEntry allows individuals to log their entries and exits from various locations, including shopping malls, restaurants, coffee shops, etc., via QR codes. Those who downloaded and enabled the TraceTogether application on their smartphones can also share detailed contact history for contact tracing purposes, as individuals with TraceTogether in close proximity will each log an entry on their phones. Geographic information system (GIS) analysis of places that cases have visited provides an additional layer of information as well. These technologies enabled a more rapid and accurate mapping of contacts to reduce the chances of missing out on contacts and decrease the time taken to quarantine contacts. Any contact who reported being symptomatic was immediately sent to a hospital for further evaluation. Contacts who were well were then placed under quarantine or daily phone surveillance and monitored closely. To ensure that close contacts were not subclinical cases, entry and exit PCR swab tests were performed at the start and end of a 14-day quarantine. A "ring" was thus drawn around each confirmed case to contain any transmission and prevent further spread.

A similar strategy was implemented for persons on Stay-Home Notice (SHN). These are individuals who had just entered Singapore and thus may have potentially been infected while overseas. Upon entering Singapore, all travellers were placed on SHN. Those from lower-risk countries with suitable residences were allowed to serve their SHN in their place of residence while others from higher-risk countries had to serve their SHN in dedicated facilities to ensure isolation for 14 days. Towards the end of SHN, individuals are required to undergo a PCR swab test.

When clusters of cases were detected, additional regional screening was performed to minimise the time for case detection and isolation, due to the suspicion of extended spread. For example, when a cluster of cases was detected involving several residences in a geographical vicinity, screening was extended to other households, eateries and shops along the road due to the possibility of the residents having frequented these other places. In another case involving two households in a Housing and Development Board (HDB) flat, screening was offered to all individuals living on the same stack as the affected units.

Active surveillance

Several groups were identified to undergo active surveillance due to an increased risk of infection among themselves or to others. These groups include foreign workers residing in dormitories, frontline workers, nursing home staff, and pre-school staff. Due to the large congregated settings that foreign workers who reside in dormitories are exposed to, the risk of rapid spread is high, thus routine regular testing at 14-day intervals was performed. This would also minimise the risk of spread to the general community as foreign workers continue working in the community. Frontline workers, nursing home staff, and pre-school staff were also placed on active surveillance to minimise the risk of nursing home clusters and healthcare clusters as these staff members interact with patients or at-risk individuals. Cases detected via active surveillance were mostly asymptomatic and found to be past infections through positive serology tests.

Other surveillance systems

Complementary to the active surveillance, Singapore tapped on pre-existing surveillance systems such as those monitoring influenza-like-illness or acute respiratory illness. General Practitioners (GP) or polyclinics may randomly swab selected individuals with relevant symptoms. During usual times, these swabs are tested for influenza. With the COVID-19 pandemic, additional testing for SARS-CoV-2 was also performed. Modelling based on these data provided indications of the numbers of undetected cases within the community, which suggest the actual extent of spread.

PCR swab testing was also performed on all patients with severe illness or death from possibly infectious causes (SIDPIC).

Enablers for case detection

The initial case detection strategies relied mostly on the suspect case definition, ringfencing around confirmed cases, and tapping on pre-existing surveillance of influenza-like-illness. Testing was subsequently extended to high-risk groups such as close contacts and incoming travellers, to enable early identification of cases.

The additional case detection strategies outlined in the previous section were implemented in a stepwise manner and gradually expanded as Singapore's testing capacity increased. This required an increase in testing resources such as PCR swabs and clinical laboratory facilities, trained healthcare workers to perform the swabs, as well as adequate personal protective equipment (PPE) to protect the frontline staff performing the tests.

To expand its testing capacity, Singapore took a multi-pronged approach. PCR swabs and testing reagents were procured from multiple sources while local researchers worked to develop new methods of swab production through 3D-printing and injection moulding. The network of Public Health Preparedness Clinics (PHPCs), which consists of selected private GP clinics was re-activated, providing easy access to healthcare providers who perform PCR swabs within the community under the SASH scheme. Individuals from other industries, which were hit by the economic downturn, were hired and trained to perform nasopharyngeal swabs to increase the personnel available and deployed to Regional Screening Centres (RSCs).

Detailed plans for testing strategy, which prioritised high-risk individuals and gradually extended to others as testing capacity was ramped up, ensured a gradual expansion of testing within resource constraints. Other methods of testing were also evaluated and deployed in various settings, including the use of pooled PCR swab testing and serology antibody testing. PCR swab tests remain the gold standard for diagnostic purposes with high sensitivity and specificity in the acute phase of the illness. Thus, Singapore continues to use PCR tests for diagnostic purposes. Together with PCR tests, serology tests have been used in certain circumstances to ensure that individuals are infection-free or have recovered before they return to work and interact with the general community. However, the utility of serology testing has been limited due to the time taken for seroconversion and the development of antibodies. Singapore continues to evaluate new testing methods as they are developed, such as sewage testing, stool testing, saliva testing, and antigen testing, to increase accessibility and availability to rapid tests and develop new case detection strategies.

Containment measures

In addition to a multi-layered case detection for early isolation of confirmed cases, effective containment also requires the rapid quarantine of close contacts who are at high risk for becoming cases and pre-emptive SHNs for travellers. Close contacts of confirmed cases are placed in quarantine for 14 days while incoming travellers are placed on SHN for 14 days. Due to knowledge on infectivity among asymptomatic individuals, a conservative period of 14 days allows adequate time for incubation during which infected cases may still test negative on PCR swab tests. With increasing evidence that a proportion of cases may remain asymptomatic or subclinical even when infected, PCR swab tests are performed towards the end of quarantine or SHN to detect these cases.

Confirmed cases were kept in isolation until they were clinically well and tested negative on PCR swab tests twice at least 24 hours apart. This was a cautious approach during the initial phase of the outbreak when knowledge on the duration of infectiousness was limited. As the outbreak progressed, global and local data suggested that patients may no longer be infective beyond 10 to 14 days of illness despite positive PCR tests. This is due to the prolonged shedding of a non-viable virus that is not related to infectivity. With the increasing evidence corroborating this finding, the de-isolation policy was reviewed to allow patients to be discharged at day 21 of illness — a conservative estimate to account for a variable duration of infectivity among different patients and to allow for adequate clinical monitoring and recovery. With the change in policy, there was no longer a need for PCR swab tests for de-isolation, allowing the redeployment of precious resources for diagnostic purposes.

Reducing importation of cases

Singapore implemented temperature screening and health declarations at borders for incoming travellers to detect febrile and unwell travellers for further evaluation to minimise the risk of transmission of COVID-19. However, the effectiveness of temperature screening is limited due to the fluctuating nature of the fever where a single time point is inadequate to detect unwell individuals. In addition, not all infected individuals may present with a febrile illness. It is also known from overseas reports that individuals may self-medicate prior to travel and thus appear afebrile at the point of entry. This measure would also fail to pick up individuals within the incubation period who would still be well.

Thus, to mitigate the spread of COVID-19 within the community, additional measures such as SHNs were issued to incoming travellers. This was initially issued to travellers from China and later gradually extended to all incoming travellers. A SHN required travellers to remain in their place of residence for 14 days, accounting for the incubation period, to minimise the risk of transmission of COVID-19 if they were infected overseas. As the risk of importation and the formation of household clusters around these cases increased, the government provided designated facilities for travellers to serve out their SHN.

As Singapore continued to identify increasing numbers of imported cases, additional border control measures were implemented, disallowing short-term visitors from landing or transiting in Singapore. Similar to SHNs, this initially involved only travellers from the epicentre of Wuhan, China, but was gradually extended to all travellers from any country as COVID-19 spread globally.

The above measures were highly effective in reducing the importation and mitigating the onwards transmission of COVID-19. With the border control measures in place from 24 March 2020, the number of imported cases gradually decreased. As Singaporeans, permanent residents and long term pass holders are still allowed entry, SHNs in designated facilities helped to mitigate onwards transmission, especially to their household members.

Reducing community transmission

A myriad of risk-calibrated policies was implemented to reduce community transmission and adjusted based on the local extent of spread (Fig. 2).

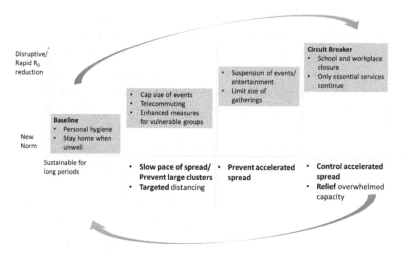

Figure 2.   Risk-calibrated social distancing measures.

Initially, the public was advised to maintain regular personal hygiene and to remain home when unwell. This reduced the risk of transmission from unwell individuals who may potentially have COVID-19, as well as to reduce the background noise from individuals with influenza or other non-COVID-19 respiratory illnesses. As community transmission was low, this placed a low burden on individuals with minimal disruption to daily life and the economy.

As local clusters started to form with suggestions of limited community transmission, restrictions on the size of events were implemented to reduce the formation of large clusters. Employers were encouraged to allow their staff to telecommute and work from home when possible so as to reduce physical interaction and transmission in the workplace. This also had the side effect of reducing crowds and close interaction among people while they were commuting on public transportation. All individuals were advised to practice safe distancing; workplaces were inspected to ensure that the work environment was modified to comply with safe distancing measures. These measures aim to slow the pace of spread and prevent the formation of large clusters. Enhanced measures were implemented for vulnerable groups such as the elderly and those residing in communal settings such as nursing homes. Similar measures were put in place among dormitories where a growing outbreak was detected, with strict enforcement of social distancing, the lockdown of affected dormitories with ongoing transmission, and systematic testing and quarantine.

With increasing community transmission, all large events were suspended, entertainment settings, such as nightclubs, with a high risk of transmission, were closed, and social gatherings were limited to small groups. Public health messaging on the need for social distancing was emphasised in various media and forms, including accessible infographics online and in public areas. These aim to prevent accelerated disease spread to ensure that our healthcare system could cope with the growing number of cases.

Despite these measures, the extent of community transmission increased. The "Circuit Breaker" (CB) was instituted on 7 April 2020, requiring all non-essential workplaces and schools to close. Individuals were required to stay home unless for essential purposes such as to purchase food or groceries or to seek medical attention. As the daily number of new cases is a lag indicator due to the incubation period, Singapore proceeded to see an increase in cases soon after the CB was instituted. This suggested the timely nature of this measure despite the extent of disruption to daily lives and the economy. The enforced social distancing from the CB was highly effective and the number of daily new cases decreased rapidly before the CB was lifted after nearly two months.

Even as community cases decreased and the situation in foreign worker dormitories came under control, social distancing remains an important measure to prevent a second wave of cases. This remains all the more important as evidence of pre-symptomatic spread suggests that even individuals who appear well may potentially be infectious. This also provided increasing evidence for mask-wearing for everyone, which was subsequently made mandatory.

Beyond social distancing measures, amendments were made to the Infectious Disease (COVID-19 Stay Orders) Regulations 2020 to legally require individuals with ARI to stay home for five days of medical leave. Due to the non-specific symptoms of COVID-19, which are clinically indistinguishable from other more common respiratory illnesses, symptomatic patients are encouraged to stay home for at least five days to minimise the risk of transmission in the event that they are infected with COVID-19. This also allowed patients to have adequate time for recovery. Those with prolonged illnesses or other forms of deterioration were then tested for COVID-19. As testing capacity increased, testing was then offered to all individuals with ARI at first presentation.

Throughout the outbreak, strong public communication was maintained through various modalities, including the traditional media, publicly located signboards and social media such as an official WhatsApp channel and Telegram chat groups. Daily situation updates kept the public apprised of the local situation, with regular press conferences held to inform the public of additional measures implemented and emphasise the public health messaging on the need for personal hygiene and safe distancing.

Frontline workers in the healthcare sector were specially monitored due to the increased risks to them and other vulnerable patients. This was also in view of the large healthcare clusters that formed during the previous 2003 SARS outbreak. Infection prevention and control measures were reviewed and reinforced to ensure adequate protection for healthcare workers. As the mode of transmission was initially unclear, healthcare workers who interacted with confirmed cases were recommended to put on full PPE, including an N95 face mask or powered air-purifying respirator (PAPR), eye protection in the form of a face shield or goggles, a gown and gloves. Healthcare workers in other areas were recommended to don various tiers of PPE based on risk levels, but minimally a medical-grade face mask. As PCR swab tests were gradually extended to the community setting where GPs perform nasopharyngeal swabs, PPE was distributed to clinics to ensure adequate protection while performing this procedure. The measures were effective, and there were no large healthcare clusters identified to date.

Conclusion

The measures outlined in this chapter will only be partially effective if utilised individually. The strategies must be implemented together to have a synergistic effect and act as a multi-layered net to address the limitations in any single measure.

References

Asadi S, Wexler AS, Cappa CD et al. (2019) Aerosol emission and superemission during human speech increase with voice loudness. Sci Rep 9:2348.

BMJ Best Practice. (2020) Coronavirus disease 2019 (COVID-19). https://best-practice.bmj.com/topics/en-us/3000168.

Byambasuren O, Cardona M, Bell K et al. (2020) Estimating the extent of asymptomatic COVID-19 and its potential for community transmission: Systematic review and meta-analysis. JAMMI 5(4):223–34. doi: 10.3138/jammi-2020-0030

Centers for Disease Control and Prevention. (2020) Interim clinical guidance for management of patients with confirmed coronavirus disease (COVID-19). https://www.cdc.gov/coronavirus/2019-ncov/hcp/clinical-guidance-management-patients.html.

Cheng PK, Wong DA, Tong LK et al. (2004) Viral shedding patterns of coronavirus in patients with probable severe acute respiratory syndrome. Lancet 363:1699–700.

Chia PY, Coleman KK, Tan YK et al. (2020) Detection of air and surface contamination by SARS-CoV-2 in hospital rooms of infected patients. Nat Commun 11:2800.

Edridge AW, Kaczorowska JM, Hoste AC et al. (2020) Coronavirus protective immunity is short-lasting. Nat Med 26:1691–93. doi: 10.1038/s41591-020-1083-1

Epidemiology Working Group for NCIP Epidemic Response, Chinese Center for Disease Control and Prevention (2020) The epidemiological characteristics of an outbreak of 2019 novel coronavirus diseases (COVID-19) in China. Zhonghua Liu Xing Bing Xue Za Zhi 41:145–51. (in Chinese)

European Centre for Disease Prevention and Control. (2020) Immune responses and immunity to SARS-CoV-2. https://www.ecdc.europa.eu/en/covid-19/latest-evidence/immune-responses

Hamner L, Dubbel P, Capron I et al. (2020) High SARS-CoV-2 attack rate following exposure at a choir practice — Skagit County, Washington, March 2020. Morb Mortal W Rep 69:606–10.

He X, Lau EHY, Wu P et al. (2020) Temporal dynamics in viral shedding and transmissibility of COVID-19. Nat Med 26:672–75.

Iwasaki A. (2020) What reinfections mean for COVID-19. Lancet Infect Dis 21(1):3–5.

Kam KQ, Yung CF, Cui L et al. (2020) A well infant with Coronavirus Disease 2019 with high viral load. Clin Infect Dis 71:847–49.

Korea Centers for Disease Control and Prevention. (2020) Findings from investigation and analysis of re-positive cases. https://www.cdc.go.kr/board/board.es?mid=&bid=0030

Lauer SA, Grantz KH, Bi Q et al. (2020) The incubation period of coronavirus disease 2019 (COVID-19) from publicly reported confirmed cases: Estimation and application. Ann Intern Med 172:577–82.

Le Bert N, Tan AT, Kunasegaran K et al. (2020) SARS-CoV-2-specific T cell immunity in cases of COVID-19 and SARS, and uninfected controls. Nature 584:457–62.

Liu Y, Gayle AA, Wilder-Smith A, Rocklöv J. (2020) The reproductive number of COVID-19 is higher compared to SARS coronavirus. J Travel Med 27(2).

McIntosh K. (2020) Coronavirus disease 2019 (COVID-19): Epidemiology, virology, and prevention. UpToDate.

Meyerowitz-Katz G, Merone L. (2020) A systematic review and meta-analysis of published research data on COVID-19 infection-fatality rates. Int J Infect Dis 101:138–48. doi: 10.1016/j.ijid.2020.09.1464

Morawska L, Milton DK. (2020) It is time to address airborne transmission of COVID-19. Clin Infect Dis 71(9):2311–13.

National Centre for Infectious Diseases and the Chapter of Infectious Disease Physicians, Academy of Medicine, Singapore. (2020) Position statement on period of infectivity to inform strategies for de-isolation for COVID-19 patients. 23 May. https://www.ncid.sg/Documents/Period%20of%20Infectivity%20Position%20 Statementv2.pdf

National Centre for Infectious Diseases. (2020) Three national-level seroepidemi-ological studies to determine level of COVID-19 infection in Singapore. 29 April. https://www.ncid.sg/News-Events/News/Pages/Three-national-level-seroepidemiological-studies-to-determine-level-of-COVID-19-infection-in-Singapore.aspx

Ng D, Klepac P, Liu Y, Prem K, Jit M, Eggo RM. (2020) Age-dependent effects in the transmission and control of COVID-19 epidemics. Nat Med **26**:1205–11.

Ong SWX, Tan YK, Chia PY *et al.* (2020) Air, surface environmental, and personal protective equipment contamination by Severe Acute Respiratory Syndrome Coronavirus 2 (SARS-CoV-2) from a symptomatic patient. *JAMA* **323**:1610–2.

Pollán M, Pérez-Gómez B, Pastor-Barriuso R *et al.* (2020) Prevalence of SARS-CoV-2 in Spain (ENE-COVID): A nationwide, population-based seroepidemi-ological study. Lancet. doi: https://doi.org/10.1016/S0140-6736(20)31483-5

Pung R, Chiew CJ, Young BE *et al.* (2020) Investigation of three clusters of COVID-19 in Singapore: Implications for surveillance and response measures. *Lancet* **395**:1039–46.

Rajgor DD, Lee MH, Archuleta S, Bagdasarian N, Quek SC. (2020) The many esti-mates of the COVID-19 case fatality rate. *Lancet Infect Dis* **20**:776–77.

Wang Y, Tong J, Qin Y *et al.* (2020) Characterization of an asymptomatic cohort of SARS-COV-2 infected individuals outside of Wuhan, China. *Clin Infect Dis* **71**(16):2132–38.

Wei WE, Li Z, Chiew CJ *et al.* (2020) Presymptomatic transmission of SARS-CoV-2 — Singapore, January 23–March 16, 2020. *Morb Mortal W Rep* **69**:411–15.

Wölfel R, Corman VM, Guggemos W *et al.* (2020) Virological assessment of hospi-talized patients with COVID-2019. *Nature* **581**:465–69.

World Health Organization. (2020) Criteria for releasing COVID-19 patients from iso-lation. 17 June. https://www.who.int/publications/i/item/criteria-for-releasing-covid-19-patients-from-isolation

World Health Organization. (2020) Report of the WHO-China Joint Mission on Corona-virus Disease 2019 (COVID-19). 28 February. https://www.who.int/docs/default-source/coronaviruse/who-china-joint-mission-on-covid-19-final-report.pdf

World Health Organization. (2020) Transmission of SARS-CoV-2: Implications for infection prevention precautions. https://www.who.int/publications/i/item/modes-of-transmission-of-virus-causing-covid-19-implications-for-ipc-precaution-recommendations.

Young BE, Ong SWX, Kalimuddin S *et al*. (2020) Epidemiologic features and clinical course of patients infected with SARS-CoV-2 in Singapore. JAMA **323**:1488–94.

Yung CF, Kam KQ, Chong CY *et al*. (2020) Household transmission of Severe Acute Respiratory Syndrome Coronavirus 2 from adults to children. *J Pediatr* **225**:249–51.

Zheng S, Fan J, Yu F *et al*. (2020) Viral load dynamics and disease severity in patients infected with SARS-CoV-2 in Zhejiang province, China, January–March 2020: Retrospective cohort study. *BMJ* **369**:m1443.

Singapore's Laboratory Response to the COVID-19 Pandemic

Raymond Lin Tzer Pin[a]

Events — Immediate Response and Timeline. Expanding Testing to Laboratories

The laboratory started the new year on Thursday, 2 Jan 2020, with news that a cluster of unexplained atypical pneumonia cases linked to a market in Wuhan had been reported to the World Health Organization (WHO). Although details were scant, it felt like we had a situation just like the beginning of the SARS outbreak in 2003. We prepared our laboratory testing panels for respiratory pathogens, including the Film Array respiratory panel and PCRs for influenza, MERS, SARS and pan-coronavirus. In particular, we reviewed our pan-coronavirus assay to ensure that it could detect members of the beta coronaviruses to which SARS and SARS-like viruses belonged. Our testing protocol for suspect cases was implemented on 6 January.

On Sunday, 12 January, the Chinese Center for Disease Control and Prevention (China CDC) released the first whole genome sequences of the novel coronavirus to the Global Initiative on Sharing all Influenza Data (GISAID) platform. The National Public Health Laboratory (NPHL) designed a PCR assay for the "2019-nCoV" (as it was called before the virus was named SARS-CoV-2) and this was implemented on 13 January. This was ten

[a] Director, National Public Health Laboratory, NCID.

days before the arrival of the first case in Singapore. As positive controls were not available yet, we continued performing our pan-coronavirus assay. The NPHL assay targeted the *orf1ab*, S and N regions. Coincidentally the China CDC test protocol released some days later also targeted the same regions. Later, the NPHL decided to use mainly the *orf1ab* and N targets for routine testing. On 17 January, Charité Hospital, Berlin, released a test protocol based on a modification of their old SARS PCR, targeting RdRP and E regions ("Charité Protocol") and this was adopted by the laboratory at the Singapore General Hospital (SGH). The synthetic positive controls for the NPHL assay arrived a week later, and on 22 January, the validation of the NPHL assay was complete. The first case in Singapore presented to the SGH on 23 January, and samples taken from the case tested positive on both the SGH "Charité" assay and the NPHL assay. A second sample was obtained to confirm the result, and genome sequencing was performed to confirm the sequence.

Following the first case, the pan-coronavirus assay was dropped. All previous suspect cases since 2 January were re-tested with the 2019-nCoV assay to ensure we did not miss any cases. In addition to the suspect cases, we started to test samples submitted under influenza-like illness surveillance and the SIDPIC (severe illness and death from possibly infectious causes) programme. The SIDPIC programme is a hospital-based sentinel surveillance programme to investigate cases of unexplained deaths and critical illness to identify possible emerging infections caused by novel pathogens.

Over several weeks following our first case, the eight public hospital laboratories with molecular diagnostic capabilities implemented COVID-19 PCR testing. The NPHL assay method was shared with the laboratories as a basis to implement laboratory-developed tests. A local test kit, Fortitude 2.0, was developed by the Agency for Science, Technology and Research (A*STAR) in collaboration with Tan Tock Seng Hospital and was granted Provisional Authorisation by the Health Sciences Authority (HSA). Eventually, other commercial test kits were also granted Provisional Authorisation. With the wider availability of commercial test kits and the increasing test capacity required to test more subjects, such as patients admitted under the enhanced pneumonia surveillance (EPS) programme in hospitals, migrant workers at dormitories and residents of nursing homes, the private laboratories also joined the network of COVID-19 PCR testing laboratories.

For laboratories to offer COVID-19 testing, they first had to be licensed clinical laboratories under the Private Hospitals and Medical Clinics Act. In addition, the Ministry of Health (MOH) also required laboratories to send the first ten positive and ten negative tests to the NPHL for parallel testing to make a recommendation to approve the laboratory for COVID-19 testing. Requirements to ensure compliance with supervision, quality and biosafety standards were eventually incorporated into Terms and Conditions for COVID-19 testing.

Most of the SARS-CoV-2 PCR testing was performed using standard real-time PCR on commonly used machines. By May 2020, other proprietary systems with special features were also implemented, such as machines with sample-to-result automation and cartridge-based PCR systems enabling turnaround times of under one hour that could be deployed to lower complexity laboratories. A local test kit for direct PCR with RNA concentration and extraction, Resolute 2.0, was developed to address the shortage of extraction kits. However, in time, alternative extraction machines were obtained by most laboratories to run with their standard PCR assays.

Other Laboratory Functions — Virus Isolation, NGS, Serology

The NPHL performed virus isolation as part of its public health functions. This was to enable whole replicating viruses to be available for high-quality genome sequencing and to make the virus available to researchers. Virus isolation was performed in the BSL3 laboratory at the MD6 building at the National University of Singapore (NUS) and later at the BSL3 laboratory in NCID. The staff at NUS had trained NPHL staff in the use of the BSL3 laboratory in 2019 and the NPHL was operating in one of the NUS BSL3 modular laboratories. The staff of the NUS Department of Microbiology and Immunology and the NUS BSL3 committee helped to facilitate the rapid and effective set up of virus isolation facilities for SARS-CoV-2. The National Centre for Infectious Diseases (NCID) BSL3 laboratory had recently been built and started operating in late 2020.

The NPHL performed whole-genome sequencing (WGS) on isolates and from specimens directly. For clinical specimens, this required adoption of enrichment methods to enable more complete and higher-quality sequences to be obtained. The Bioinformatics Institute (BII) of A*STAR helped with the analysis of WGS sequences from Singapore. The BII also played a key role in helping the GISAID curate and maintain the database of sequences from around the world. The GISAID is the main global repository of SARS-CoV-2 sequences. Duke-NUS also performed WGS on their virus isolates from research subjects and the NPHL played a coordinating role to link the genetic data to the epidemiology investigations conducted by the MOH.

Antibody testing (serology) had no role to play in the routine diagnosis of acute illness for COVID-19 and the MOH issued a circular to all medical practitioners providing advice on the proper use of rapid antibody test kits. However, by May, antibody-testing was considered an important tool for establishing epidemiology links, resolving uncertain diagnoses, determining prevalence in various subpopulations, and monitoring seroprevalence. In particular, serology was used to determine control strategies to guide migrant worker dormitories in resuming normal functions while reducing the risk of further outbreaks. This was helped by the availability of reliable test kits for autoanalysers using chemiluminescent bead technology, already in use in clinical laboratories. In addition, a test for neutralising antibodies developed by Duke-NUS using a novel competitive binding approach was commercialised and called "cPass". cPass was evaluated and deployed by the NPHL to assist MOH investigations and to support seroprevalence studies.

Collaborations with Research Laboratories

The NPHL and Duke-NUS made available virus isolates for investigations into SARS-CoV-2 virulence and biological properties animal model studies as well as diagnostic and therapeutic approaches. Other hospital laboratories also worked with their respective research groups to make available their expertise and facilities to evaluate new diagnostic test kits. The research laboratories performed studies on immune profiles and other factors related to SARS-CoV-2 pathogenicity. Various groups developed approaches to antibody, antigen and nucleic acid detection. Therapeutic and vaccine studies by research groups also relied on collaboration with front-line laboratories.

Rapid and Innovative Tests. Evaluation Systems. Diagnostics Panels

There were many proposals from commercial and research entities to provide novel devices for diagnostic purposes. While HSA authorisation was required for eventual deployment as clinical tests, we were faced with the question of whether some new methods, groups or products were promising enough to be supported by funding, advice or collaboration with potential end-users. At the NCID, various proposals were collated and assessed by the diagnostics screening team, and its comments and recommendations were forwarded to a diagnostics assessment panel chaired by the Chief Health Scientist of MOH and comprised other scientists with domain expertise in applications of innovative science. Later, a Technology Evaluation and Implementation Unit was formed by MOH to perform horizon scanning and evaluation of new technologies.

Patient Groups — Suspects, ILI, ARI, Enhanced, Dorm, PUQ, Evacuation Flights, Surge Capacity

Even though standard real-time PCR remained the main testing method, the types of patients tested changed over the course of the pandemic. Initially, testing was directed at suspect cases with symptoms, including enhanced surveillance of those with pneumonia and gradually broadening criteria for acute respiratory infections (ARIs). Clearance swabs for hospitalised patients took up a substantial volume of testing. Testing of passengers on evacuation flights from Wuhan, persons under quarantine (PUQs), nursing home residents, contacts of confirmed cases, and migrant workers in dormitories were other groups that presented different challenges. In asymptomatic subjects, e.g., those screened in contact tracing investigations, the risk of false-positives was higher than in clinically-suspect cases. Those who had been infected for some time often had borderline PCR readings or just one target positive in a test kit with two or three targets. These often required repeat testing or assessment by another sample, and even then, the conclusion was not always definitive. The use of antibody tests helped form part of the clinical assessment. Dormitory cases often had high positivity rates, and care was needed to prevent cross-contamination of PCR laboratories. For some patients, multiple tests and assessment over time was the only way to make a final assessment of whether the patient was infected. To support the reopening of the economy, institutions and services, mass screening of essential workers and those working with vulnerable groups required new laboratory testing approaches. We introduced pooled testing by combining multiple swabs in one UTM container. In 2021, we began seeing more cases or re-infection, often with virus variants, as well as some vaccine breakthrough infections. Theses investigations required a laboratory testing with PCR, virus isolation, whole genome sequencing and quantitative serial serology.

Surge Capacity. Our pandemic planning for influenza had a targeted laboratory testing capacity of 2,200 PCR tests per day. This was based on our 2009 experience and modelling that indicated that once the infection was widespread, mitigation would take place and only high-risk patients needed to be tested. However, SARS-CoV-2 has proven highly transmissible, yet transmission could be interrupted with intensive testing and contact tracing. So our testing strategy expanded and needed to be sustained to contain the infection, to limit the number infected to "flatten the curve", to protect vulnerable groups and, in the coming months, to find a way to re-open society and the economy while ensuring that healthcare resources are not overwhelmed. These objectives meant expanding the testing capacity to 8,800 PCR tests a day, achieved by our public and private clinical laboratories. As of mid-July, we have conducted more than 1 million PCR tests, and our overall test rate is one of the highest in the world. Nevertheless, the strategies planned require a test capacity of more than 40,000 tests per day. A separate and dedicated COVID-19 testing laboratory was set up, and plans for further ramping up required challenges to be met with respect to accuracy, biosafety, logistics, informatics, manpower and supervision.

Reagent Supplies and Diversification

After the pandemic reached Europe and the United States (US), supply shortages became an issue. This affected the supply of swabs and UTM containers first, followed by RNA concentration and extraction kits for automated machines. Alternative suppliers were sourced from Korea, China and elsewhere. This alleviated the shortage to a large extent. However, challenges faced with the diversity of sources included: quality of manufacturing, unsuitable specifications, sub-optimal performance, incompatibility with current tests, and user acceptance. We are endeavouring to develop local manufacturing for the full range of supplies, and in some areas have already been relatively successful, e.g., PCR test kits. The role of ALPS, Temasek Foundation and the Economic Development Board in the procurement efforts have been invaluable in preserving our laboratory capacity.

Appointments — Referral Laboratory, Experts, Consultation

The NPHL was appointed as a WHO referral laboratory for COVID-19 testing, and we participated in a weekly meetings of the WHO Expert Panel in Laboratory Testing as well as a separate groups on re-infection. We have tested specimens from members states in the Western Pacific Region and provided informal advice and opinions on laboratory issues. The NPHL also participates in the Regional Public Health Laboratory Network in this region, under the auspices of the Global Health Security Agenda, led by Thailand. We have helped facilitate the sharing of information and experience among member states during this pandemic.

Evolving needs

With the expanding numbers and indications for testing, the NPHL helps in the investigation of problem cases like discordant results and persistent PCR positives. It also evaluates the strategic application of new tests like new serology methods.

We are also assessing new proposals using next-generation sequencing technology for high throughput diagnostic testing. Local researchers developed rapid tests based on molecular capture, isothermal reactions, and other formats that still need analytical and clinical validation.

The challenge of potential mass testing in asymptomatic population groups have raised questions of alternative specimens like saliva. This is a challenging issue as the published data have been conflicting and inconclusive.

We also saw more cases with borderline PCR results that may be false-positives or represent the tail-end of an infection. These may be seen in asymptomatic subjects with low pre-test likelihood. On the other hand, previously infected migrant workers may show up weeks or months later with positive PCR results, usually with a low viral RNA load. It is not clear when these might represent re-infection over time.

Serology increasingly plays a role, together with PCR, in assessing the extent of clusters and resolving cases that are borderline or have possible prolonged shedding. Seroprevalence studies in various population groups will track the spread of the virus in the community.

The large number of tests done by many laboratories of varying experience in PCR testing means we have to deal with more suspected cases of false-positives or false-negatives. These could be due to many errors, whether human or machine, calibration, non-compliant practice or contamination.

Widespread testing in the community also requires a standardised logistic and information flow, from the point of specimen collection, labelling and transport, to specimen receipt, processing and reporting. The information technology agencies have designed systems to meet these needs. Good IT support and systems are integral to laboratory response to this pandemic.

By early 2021, the world was faced with questions relating to virus variants of concern, re-infection, monitoring vaccine effectiveness and vaccine breakthrough infections. The NPHL conducted serological investigations and increased its gene sequencing capabilities to help in assessment and inform new policies. Other challenges include strategies to determine immunity in travellers, and finding suitable tests to allow opening up of international travel, recovering of economic activity and return to more live social events.

7 Clinical Care and the COVID-19 Outbreak

Shawn Vasoo, Bernard Thong, Margaret Soon, Ang Hou, Albert Tan, Tan Hui Ling and Benjamin Ho

The COVID-19 pandemic has been unprecedented in multiple ways. SARS-CoV-2, the third described zoonotic novel coronavirus, was unlike its predecessors SARS-CoV and MERS-CoV in its emergence and dramatic worldwide spread, its mode of spread (asymptomatic and pre-symptomatic transmission) and varied spectrum of disease, from completely asymptomatic to mild, then severe (Lee and Vasoo, 2020). These have challenged traditional paradigms of clinical management, including case identification and screening, contact tracing and public health measures. In this chapter we review key facets of the pandemic response in the clinical care of COVID-19, focusing primarily on the ramping up of clinical services at the National Centre for Infectious Diseases (NCID), a 14-storey purpose-built isolation facility, and Tan Tock Seng Hospital (TTSH), including operational considerations, a broad overview of the clinical response of the healthcare system in Singapore, and an overview of planning and considerations for COVID-19 therapeutics.

Overview

As of 15 July 2020, Singapore saw a total of 46,878 COVID-19 cases, of which 128 (0.3%) required ICU admission, and 92% had recovered and were discharged. As of 30 June, a total of 7,720 COVID-19 patients have been admitted to the NCID since the first case of COVID-19 was identified in Singapore.

This chapter presents a comprehensive overview of pandemic response in patient care areas, which include a dedicated screening centre, ambulatory clinic, inpatient wards, intensive care units, etc.

NCID Screening Centre

The NCID Screening Centre (SC) is a purpose-built facility designed for mass screening and other related activities (e.g., vaccination) in outbreaks and is located at the basement 1 level of the NCID.

Physical infrastructure

The SC has a total floor area of 4,980 m² and is equipped with infrastructure and equipment that allows it to function as a "one-stop suite" of services (Fig. 1) — a sorting area, triage zones, waiting areas, consult, procedure

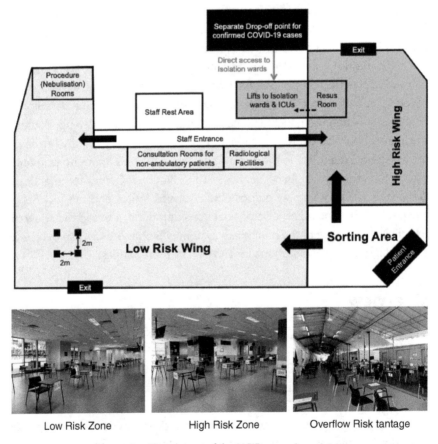

Figure 1. Floor layout of the NCID screening centre.

Table 1.   Facilities within the NCID screening centre.

Facilities	Low Risk Area	High Risk Area	Overflow Tentage
Consult/Procedure Rooms	8	6	4
Negative Pressure/Isolation Rooms	4	1	—
Resuscitation Rooms	1	1	—
X-ray	2	1	1 (portable)
Pharmacy	1	1	2 (medicine store)
Waiting and In-seat Assessment Areas (Total capacity: 110, if seats spaced 2 m apart; 204 if spaced 1.5 m apart)	4	1	4

and resuscitation rooms, diagnostic imaging, and an on-site pharmacy. The SC is divided functionally into "low risk areas" and "high risk areas" into which attendees may be sorted, based on epidemiologic and clinical risks. At the height of the COVID-19 pandemic, the capacity of the SC was increased by setting up overflow tentages around and adjacent to the SC, which increased its capacity (Table 1).

Infection control and PPE

The air in the SC undergoes a change of 12 times per hour, is HEPA-filtered, and undergoes UV treatment. Staff rest areas (pantry, toilets/showers, masking rooms) are maintained at positive pressure in relation to the screening areas. The staff entering the area change into scrubs and don an N95 mask in a masking room and then proceed to a dedicated area to don the rest of their personal protective equipment (PPE) (the entire ensemble comprising of an N95 mask, eye protection, an AAMI-level 4 equivalent gown, and gloves, also known as "full PPE") before they can enter the "hot-zone", with the process occurring in reverse when exiting the area. To facilitate contact tracing activities should the need arise, the SC is also equipped with CCTVs and transponders for tag-based real-time location service tracking, which allow accurate monitoring of staff and patients and their interactions.

Manpower and workflows

A total of ~168 staff per shift are required to man the SC when at capacity (without overflow tentage) (Table 2), which is 22 trolley beds and 99 ambu-

Table 2. Screening centre manpower per shift when at capacity.

Family Group	No. of Staff
Medical	26
Nursing	60
Radiology	7
Pharmacy	8
Security	13
Patient Service Assistants	11
Operations (Logistics)	6
Operations (Data Management)	2
Housekeeping	22
Portering	13
Total (per Shift)	168

latory patients when chairs are spaced 2 metres apart, or a seating capacity of 181 when chairs are spaced 1.5 metres apart, at any point (Table 1). Workflows are in place to ensure efficient ingress, sorting, triage, assessment and disposition of patients as well as to ensure safety and adherence to strict infection control throughout the patient journey (including safe distancing and masking of all patients). Self-guided questionnaires were placed on patient's tables to enhance the efficient collection of epidemiologic risks and clinical features during the consultation.

COVID-19 Ramp-up and Operations

Patient attendances for suspect COVID screening at TTSH Emergency Department (ED) progressively increased in January 2020. As part of heightened alert and outbreak readiness, the NCID outbreak team (NCID Nursing and NCID Operations) kick-started the physical set-up of the SC (bare during "peace-time") on the week beginning 20 January, which lasted for a week. The set-up included IT equipment, medical equipment and medical consumables.

Because TTSH ED was nearing maximum capacity, it was decided on 28 January to divert and centralise all COVID screening to the SC. The SC was activated and operationalised on 29 January, and was initially led and run by the NCID outbreak team with contingency manpower injected in the first two days by both the Emergency Department (ED) and Infectious Diseases Department specialists, and ED/NCID Nursing, so as to allow TTSH's Division of Surgery a three-day lead time to degrade "business-as-usual" (BAU) activities (i.e., non-critical/urgent services and appointments) and release manpower to support and sustain 24/7 operations. Within the NCID, staff members from public health units dropped all non-critical non-urgent work and underwent just-in-time training on mask fitting, PPE ground orientation and operations briefing, so as to fill and augment ground operations and other roles such as sorting, security enforcement and patient wayfinding. Due to the forward projections and rapid tempo of the COVID-19 situation, the SC started operations thus started at H+24, instead of H+72.

At H+72, SC operations were transitted to and helmed by the ED, with medical manpower largely supplied by the Division of Surgery, whose BAU activities were ramped down. Based on screening/attendance volumes, manpower needs were adjusted dynamically.

Daily attendance increased to ~200 in February. There was a need to prepare for surge capacity. In close discussion with Infection Control, it was decided that seating could be reduced safely from 2 m to 1.5 m apart, which increased the capacity to 178. A drawer plan to overflow attendees to Clinic J (with J Clinic BAU decanted to an alternative site) was reviewed but decided against by Infection Control and Engineering due to concerns over the air regime provision in the J clinic area outside of the Special Precautions Area (SPA). To further increase capacity, open and well-ventilated tentage areas would be set up adjacent to the SC to increase the COVID-19 screening and holding capacity.

Upon approval from the relevant authorities, the vendor set up the tentage swiftly within a week, and the team operationalised it on 20 March, with an added capacity of 61. This was about the time when COVID-19 was fast spreading in dormitories, with daily attendances fluctuating from 200 to 500 plus.

Month	Total Attendance
January	281
February	4,669
March	8,466
April	7,671
May	5,373
June	4,035
Total	**30,495**

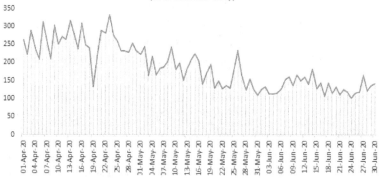

Daily Attendance at NCID SC
(as of 2359hrs daily)

Figure 2. Monthly (January–June 2020) and daily screening centre attendances (April–June 2020)

On 17 March, with a change in the Ministry of Health (MOH)'s suspect case definition, the attendance reached 493 for the day and a queue extended to the ambulance bay. Clinic J's SPA was activated to help clear the load as patients were kept waiting for more than four hours. With a change in MOH strategy to do swab-and-hold before decant or transfer, some patients had long wait-times in the SC (sometimes overnight, while awaiting results or conveyance), thus limiting capacity.

Therefore another tentage was operationalised as a holding area on 24 April with a capacity for 51 persons. The first tentage was also extended to create a holding area, with an added capacity of 71. By this time, the total capacity of the SC and tentages was 361 at 1.5 m apart.

At the height of the pandemic, daily attendances averaged between 200–300 per day. However, a maximum of 523 attendances in a single day was realised on 23 March. Figure 2 details the attendances per month at the SC from January to June.

Key lessons

- Clear zoning and workflows are important for patient and staff safety, besides PPE.
- Both physical infrastructure and manpower planning should take into account scalability (ramping up and down) at different phases of the outbreak response, as well as local situational changes.

Ambulatory Clinic — The Special Precautions Area (SPA) and Clinic J

The Special Precautions Area (SPA) in Clinic J is a dedicated area to manage outpatients who have suspected or confirmed novel (and possibly airborne) infectious diseases.

Physical infrastructure

Functionally, pre-pandemic, the SPA had two areas (or "airborne" and "contact" precautions area, with two and three negative pressure rooms, respectively), although the SPA functioned as one area for the evaluation and follow-up of persons with suspected or confirmed COVID-19 or other airborne diseases during the pandemic.

Infection control and PPE

The SPA is maintained at a negative pressure in relation to the rest of the clinic area; air handling is separate, with 12 air changes per hour. The SPA area is equipped with CCTVs and has a registration/queue system, and all staff members have real-time locating system (RTLS) tags (these were later extended to outpatients too) to facilitate contact tracing activities if required.

Manpower and workflows

The SPA area is staffed by two to four residents/medical officers (junior doctors) under the supervision of one or more Infectious Diseases consultants, depending on the workload. Staff enter and exit the area via dedicated donning and doffing areas, which are separate, to prevent cross-contamination. The SPA waiting area seats persons under evaluation (who are also given masks) at a distance of 1.5 to 2 m, resulting in a seating capacity of 45 if individuals are paced 1.5 m apart.

Ramp-up

The SPA operates under the Infectious Diseases Specialist Outpatient Clinic J. From February 2020, BAU work was scaled down by approximately 50% and only essential ID services, such as ED referrals, HIV first visits, poorly controlled HIV infection or those newly initiated on therapy and infection exposure management, were prioritised. Additional manpower (medical, nursing and patient service assistants) were also redeployed within Clinic J to the SPA to support clinical visits related to COVID-19. This included the evaluation of patients with acute respiratory infections (ARIs) fulfilling the prevalent MOH suspect case criterion and supporting referrals from the MOH for public health — "swab and serology procedures" for persons under quarantine or epidemiologic/clinical investigations for close contacts and mass screening (e.g., "pooled positives" investigations). The SPA saw a total of 858 swabs, and/or serology attendances between April to June 2020, up from 33 between January to March (Table 3).

Given the need for proper resource allocation and that patients who have recovered from acute COVD-19 may have residual sequelae (and are therefore non-infectious) but need to be followed-up are seen in the general area in Clinic J.

Clinic J is also anchored by the Convalescent Plasma therapy screening clinic, co-led by Haematology and Infectious Diseases. A total of 133 screening visits were actualised between March to June 2020.

Since February 2020, Clinic J has scaled down its BAU (including multi-specialty services) by approximately 50%, and the extension site Day Treatment Centre was closed to consolidate all manpower and services at Clinic J to cope with the growing COVID-19 workload. To ensure continuity of care during the outbreak, blood and procedural appointments for all BAU patients were retained, and clinicians would review the test results before providing them with follow-up plans, i.e., scheduling or deferring their next appointment.

COVID-19 services at Clinic J mainly comprise referrals from the SC and suspect/confirmed COVID-19 cases discharged from hospital wards for ID follow-up at Clinic J. With increasing attendances at the SC and number of confirmed cases admitted in the NCID, a surge in referrals to Clinic J ensued. Several measures were implemented as part of the efforts to manage the increasing referrals. Firstly, with the Infection Control endorsement, the safety margin of seating distance in the SPA in Clinic J was reduced from 2 m to 1.5 m, increasing the total capacity to 45 at any one point in time. More manpower (medical, nursing and PSA) was also redeployed within Clinic J to the SPA to manage the increased workload and reduce the turnaround time. Clinic J also supports MOH public health functions through swab and serology procedures for the entry and exit of persons under quarantine (PUQs) from Government Quarantine Facilities (GQFs), epidemiology investigations for close contacts and pooled positives investigations.

While supporting the above COVID-19 functions, it is also critical to segregate COVID-19 suspects from all other ID conditions requiring isolation and to optimise the use of Clinic J spaces without compromising clinical safety. As such, Clinic J overall workflows were consistently reviewed and enhanced with the evolving situation and better understanding of COVID-19. With the Infection Control assessment and endorsement, all suspect COVID-19 patients were seen in the SPA while recovered COVID-19 patients (>21 days of illness) were seen in Cluster 2. BAU patients presenting with

Table 3.   SPA attendance for COVID-19 cases.

Isolation Precaution	Respiratory
Total Isolation Cases	1853
Percentage of Total Cases	98.4%
Percentage of Cases Admitted	4%
Conditions	Review of suspect, confirmed and swab-and-sent-home (SASH) COVID-19 cases; enhanced surveillance for COVID-19; MOH referrals for swab and serology

* Data from 1 April to 30 June 2020.

ARI symptoms or fulfilling the suspect criteria for COVID-19 would also be isolated in the SPA for further assessment. Amidst the COVID-19 outbreak, Clinic J has been managing a dengue surge since May 2020. A total of 645 dengue visits were actualised between April and June, up from 235 between January and March.

Since the Circuit Breaker (CB), Clinic J is progressing to a recovery phase with plans to resume deferred BAU services with the help of technology, i.e., teleconsultation, while maintaining its current workload of BAUs, COVID-19 and dengue outbreak.

Key lessons

- Outpatient areas, especially Infectious Diseases clinics or specialties that may evaluate patients with COVID-19 or other airborne-transmitted diseases should have designated isolation rooms, scaled to capacity-required, and ideally with negative-pressure and a separately handled air-regime.

Inpatients — General Wards and ICU

Physical infrastructure

The NCID has 330 inpatient beds across 17 wards in the following configurations — 38 negative pressured ICU beds, four High Level Isolation Unit beds and 288 negative pressured general isolation beds. These general isolation beds are in isolation rooms with anterooms, isolation rooms without anterooms, and multi-bed cohort cubicles. The NCID is also designed for scalability. Each of the isolation rooms can accommodate an extra bed, increasing the total number of beds to 586. Air handling is separate for each isolation room, with 12 air changes per hour.

Ramp-up

Since its opening in December 2018, the NCID operates a total of four Infectious Diseases Wards (80 beds), while TTSH operates three isolation wards (60 beds). TTSH and the NCID jointly operate eight ICU and two High

Dependency beds. When reports of the coronavirus emerged in January 2020, the first Outbreak ward (20 beds) was activated on 6 January to isolate patients with fever, ARIs and travel history to Wuhan, China. As the number of patients admitted continued to increase, NCID decant and conversion plans kicked in. Patients in the seven non-outbreak ("peace-time") wards were decanted out of the NCID so that they could be converted from a "peace-time" function to outbreak functions. The cohort wards were naturally ventilated during "peace-time" and hence, required partition walls to be installed and converted into negative pressured rooms.

During the last week of January, three additional Outbreak wards (60 beds) were opened to admit patients. At the peak of the ramp-up, six wards (120 beds) were opened in a single day in the first week of February. During the surge in the second week of March, an additional bed was added into each isolation room to cope with the increase in hospital admissions and cohort patients with confirmed COVID-19. In April, the beds in service within the NCID exceeded 500. The number of patients admitted in February was slightly below 900, but trended up to 1,059 in March and peaked at almost 3,000 in April, before declining to approximately 1,700 in May, with numbers primarily driven by the surge in suspect and confirmed cases from the migrant worker dormitories.

To cope with the influx of confirmed cases, the capacity in NCID wards was ramped up by redeploying additional beds and equipment from TTSH. Based on the cohorting principles of COVID-19 cases, the NCID converted single-bedded negative pressure rooms to double/triple-bedded rooms by stacking in additional beds. As the NCID continued to admit more than 500 COVID-19 cases, "peace-time" wards in TTSH (Wards 7A, 7B, 7D, 11A, 11B and 11D) and Ren Ci Community Hospital (RCCH, Wards 8, 9 and 10) were also converted into COVID-19 outbreaks wards for the overflow of COVID-19 cases. The Medical Ambulatory Centre (MAC) and CDC1 Wards were converted to short-stay units for patients awaiting transfers. Decanting operations of COVID-19 patients in stable conditions to Community Care Facilities (CCFs) or Community Recovery Facilities (CRFs) helped to free up beds in NCID wards for incoming patients.

To facilitate communications with migrant worker patients who were not conversant in English, remote translation (via phone and video conferencing) were engaged and patient admission packages and advisories

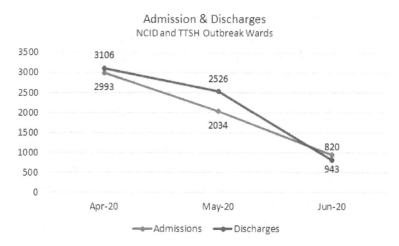

Figure 3.   Admissions and discharges in NCID and TTSH outbreak wards (April–June 2020).

were provided in their mother tongue (e.g., Bengali, Tamil, Chinese or other languages), including a link to a QR code-based video FAQ, which was filmed by the outbreak medical teams. The Medical Social Workers (MSWs) worked together with non-governmental organisations such as HealthServe to deploy COVID-19 educational videos in different languages.

With the CB measures in place, the number of inpatient admission and discharge cases from April to June 2020 decreased (Fig. 3). The peak number of admissions was realised on 22 April with 210 patients admitted, while the peak discharge number was 292 on 1 May. The first two COVID-19 deaths in Singapore were reported on 21 March. On 30 April, the campus saw the highest record of daily inflight numbers of confirmed and suspect COVID-19 cases of 900 patients.

ICU ramp-up

The NCID's ICU complement comprises 38 beds located in two wards (Ward 3E with 20 beds and Ward 3F with 18 beds). As the number of COVID-19 cases was increasing nationally, the ICU capacity needed was projected to facilitate planning and preparation. Based on a modelling assumption of 6% of all COVID-19 cases requiring the use of the ICU, a total of around 1,300 ICU beds were required, of which the campus would need to acquire 265 more. This would need coordination among multiple stakeholders and alignment with the national strategy. An ICU Coordinating Taskforce was set up to review the manpower, training and operations needed to ramp up the campus' ICU capacity. It also coordinated with the National ICU Committee overseeing ICU ramp-up across all the public hospitals in Singapore.

The ICU ramp-up can be described in the following aspects:

i. Infrastructure planning and preparation

We assessed the ICU wards available on campus before determining that in the earlier surge phase, the ICUs in the main building of TTSH used during the SARS outbreak in 2003 would have to be used again. These two ICUs (Ward 6A and Ward 6B) comprised single-bedded ICU rooms, some of which were negative pressure isolation rooms with anterooms. This was because many of the NCID beds were still occupied by COVID-19 positive patients who were yet to be decanted to community facilities, which were still being set up. Once the patients were decanted, we were able to set up four of the general wards in the NCID comprising single isolation rooms with anterooms as "ICU minus wards". The concept of ICU minus wards was nationally determined. The minimum criteria were that these wards had to be able to provide invasive mechanical ventilation with at least a transport ventilator, hemodynamic monitoring and support, and have access to intensivist support. At the NCID, conventional hemodialysis was also possible at these wards as this was factored in when planning for the building. Scalability was also factored in such that in extreme surges, some of the rooms would be able to accommodate two ICU beds instead of one.

ii. Manpower planning

Manpower was a big limiting constraint that we needed to overcome. While physical beds could still be reconfigured, the number of ICU-trained doctors, nurses and allied health professionals was small. Possible strategies included: leave freeze, deployment of all ICU-trained doctors back to the ICU from all departments, especially Respiratory Medicine, Anaesthesiology and Internal Medicine, and a rapid recall of ICU-trained doctors on rotation to other hospitals. ICU-trained nurses were recalled from all wards and augmentation of ICU-trained nurses from other hospitals was planned. Even with all this, the total number of nurses was still insufficient. An expedited conversion programme was planned by Nursing to identify nurses to be upskilled in a step-up fashion. Eligible general ward nurses were identified to undergo conversion programme to care for patients in high dependency units, and eligible high dependency unit nurses were identified to undergo conversion programme to care for patients in ICUs. Mass critical care staff to patient ratios were also established to enable consistent rostering to ensure patient safety while managing surge to ensure that patients did not come to harm due to delayed access to an ICU bed. Where manpower capacity permitted, the roster for the outbreak ICU took into consideration the added stress of working in an outbreak environment and the challenges of working with PPE, such as the additional time taken to see patients as a result of the need to don and doff PPE safely. To free up manpower to be deployed to the outbreak ICUs, the main block's ICUs were scaled down progressively with bed closures while maintaining sufficient capacity for non-outbreak demand.

iii. Staff preparation through training and drills

An education programme was established to provide doctors with a quick ICU refresher course and to train new doctors in the basics of ICU care. In addition to ICU training, training in Infection Control practices and proper use of PPE was also conducted via on-site drills in the outbreak ICUs. During the drills, staff experienced powered air-purifying respirator (PAPR) failure and learnt what to do in such an event. They also experienced eye protection goggles fogging up when inserting invasive lines and learnt how to adapt. Such preparation helped staff to become rapidly accustomed to practicing safely and effectively in the outbreak ICU environment and staff were more confident of performing their role well.

iv. Equipping of the ICU: Equipment, consumables and drugs

The ICU is heavily dependent on equipment such as ventilators, infusion pumps and physiological monitoring systems. During the outbreak and mass casualty preparation, we established a stockpile of ICU ventilators and transport ventilators for 120 ICU beds. For the COVID-19 outbreak, a national strategy was used to procure additional ventilators and equipment for all the ICUs in the country. Similarly, rapid and aggressive procurement of consumables was also started early in the outbreak. Due to supply chain disruption, drug shortages were also anticipated and a drug conservation project at the hospital level was started. In the operating theatre, a system for the safe sharing of critical drugs such as propofol and atracurium was established. Drug substitution guidelines were established, and regular monitoring of drug utilisation and drug stock commenced.

v. Coordination and triage

At full surge capacity, there would be 265 beds spread over eight locations at both the NCID and TTSH. An ICU Headquarters (ICU HQ) was established as a single point-of-contact for any ICU bed request. This provided a streamlined service that reduced confusion and delay. The ICU HQ is operated by a team of doctors supported by administrative staff. Through the use of telephonic facilitation, the ICU HQ doctor-in-charge acts as the first line triage for load balancing of the ICUs, right siting of the patient to the correct ICU depending on the acuity of the patient, and also serves as the first level of rationing according to the national ICU triage and rationing guidelines. A hospital committee consisting of clinical ethics experts, intensivists and relevant specialties such as geriatric medicine, infectious disease and general medicine was appointed for managing the complex ethical cases in ICU triage via a daily roster of three specialists for rapid consult and decision-making.

Infection control and PPE

Patients were cared for in full PPE, with powered air-purifying respirators reserved for persons requiring prolonged in-room contact time and potentially performing aerosol generating procedures. "Clean" and "dirty" staff and patient flows were kept separate as far as possible for movements. Hydrogen peroxide decontamination (as indicated, e.g., for the disinfection of single rooms after a COVID-19 positive patient is discharged) and routine terminal cleaning were supported by 24/7 operations by the environmental services team to ensure rapid turnaround.

Manpower and workflows

Months of training and drills on ward activation have prepared NCID nurses to operate the first 200 beds. However, when the ramp-up continued into the second week of February, the NCID had to rely on the augmentation of nurses from TTSH. To cope with the influx of nurses who were not prepared to manage patients with infectious diseases, a crash course on Infection Control and the donning and removal of personal protective equipment (PPE) had to be put in place. On the day of deployment to the NCID, staff members were orientated to the ward and the environment. To help the nurses navigate the new environment, the nursing team within the NCID had to be re-organised. NCID nurses were re-assigned and spread across all the wards so that the deployed nurses from TTSH had a "buddy" to help them navigate the environment. To cope with the rapidly evolving information and frequent change in policies and workflows, visual cues were placed throughout the unit. Mandatory safety huddles were also to be conducted at the start of every shift. Nursing and support services were supportive on the ground operations to ramp up the NCID to its full outbreak capacity of 330 beds. In terms of medical manpower, a total of 345 senior and junior FTEs (full-time equivalent head count) were required to run up to 586 outbreak beds (including the ICU). All these manpower were supported by a total of 1,161 FTEs deployed in rotations from TTSH hospital to the NCID to augment the 687 staff based at the NCID. Additionally, at the peak of the outbreak, manpower support was also provided by other public hospitals through the MOH and deployed to the NCID — these comprised 22 medical officers/residents and 34 nurses, among other professionals from the allied health professions.

Policies and Practices, Extracorporeal Membrane Oxygenation (ECMO) Service, Multi-disciplinary Team Model

New policies and protocols had to be established rapidly, such as the awake proning protocol, prone ventilation, and the safe use of non-invasive ventilation. A national extracorporeal membrane oxygenation (ECMO) service was set up, and drills were conducted before the first patient who would require ECMO was admitted. These efforts were supported at the NCID by the National Heart Centre and the National University Hospital. We leveraged on our "peace-time" multi-disciplinary model of care to cater to the diverse patient needs. With the advent of new drugs, the presence of a dedicated on-site ICU pharmacist who attended all the ward rounds was critical to ensuring safe and optimal therapeutics. The general wards were supported by a team of pharmacists dedicated to the NCID wards. The respiratory therapists were on-site in the ICUs and part of the code blue team for the NCID wards. The medical disciplines that were heavily involved in inpatient care included Infectious Disease, with a specialist doing daily rounds and others that attended on a consult basis such as cardiology, neurology, general surgery and neurosurgery. The anaesthetists were involved in the provision of ICU care as well as managing confirmed and suspect COVID-19 cases who needed operative management.

Patient Transport and Security

Many patients require advanced imaging such as CT scans. Hence, in addition to the usual admission and discharge transfers, protocols were established for the safe transfers of these patients, with designated routes mapped out and duties for security escort clearly spelled out. Drills were conducted for ICU patient transport, so that the multi-disciplinary teams could become familiar with the transport of critically ill patients.

Grief and Bereavement Support, Palliative Care

In any outbreak, death cannot be avoided, especially in the ICU. Medical social workers (MSWs) helped patients and their next-of-kin cope with separation/isolation and bereavement by facilitating conversations and interactions via selected in-person visits or telepresence. For the Outbreak ICUs, routines such as weekly long-stayers and palliative care rounds (attended by the ICU consultant, Palliative Medicine consultant and MSW) to discuss care plans for patients and their families were established.

Recovering from Critical Illness Due to COVID-19

Many COVID-19 survivors sustain functional debilitation and experience fatigue. ICU survivors require prolonged ventilatory support. Building on the existing ICU early rehabilitation programme, physiotherapists were involved in the care of ICU patients as soon as they were hemodynamically stable. Patients were mobilised early. Dieticians provided nutritional assessment and input on enteral as well as parenteral feeding regimes via remote access. Speech therapists played a key role as many patients had swallowing impairment following prolonged intubation. General ward patients received self-help exercise booklets to enable them to take charge of their own rehabilitation. The rehabilitation physician conducted weekly multi-disciplinary rounds for patients who were de-isolated to the main TTSH ICUs and wards. The patient's entire rehabilitation journey is coordinated from hospitalisaton to discharge.

Key lessons

- Things do not exactly happen the way one may have planned. While pre-pandemic ramp-up and surge plans, including timeline and schedules, were clearly articulated, one had to be adaptable and adjust plans according to how the pandemic evolved.
- Drills and training are important to prepare the staff on what to expect. For staff members deployed to the NCID, they had to cope with many factors, from a new and unfamiliar environment to new workflows and procedures, as well as managing their fear of the disease and anxiety of the unknown. Providing opportunities for cross-training during pre-outbreaks is important in helping allay staff anxiety.
- Good communication is crucial to ensure that staff members are updated on the rapidly changing policies, procedures and workflows.

Operational Support

Underpinning all outbreak efforts is the need for very strong operational support. COVID-19 campus operations were supported by the NCID Operations Command Centre (NOCC) and Tan Tock Seng Emergency Planning. Such operational support was required for the screening centre, J Clinic, inpatient work and the Joint Call Centre (JCC). To adapt to changing outbreak situations, the NOCC worked with various agencies such as the MOH, Ministry of Manpower (MOM), and Medical Operations Taskforce

Table 5. Volume of calls related to COVID-19.

Month	Joint Call Centre (Call Volume)	TTSH Contact Centre (Call Volume)	Total (per Month)
April	2,134	1,025	**3,159**
May	1,019	256	**1,275**
June	1,284	239	**1,523**
Total	**4,437**	**1,520**	**5,957**

(MOTF) to modify and streamline workflows along with issuances of new and enhanced government policies, and coordinating admission and discharge/decant operations.

The JCC was in charge of addressing public queries and feedback related to COVID-19. All COVID-19-related calls were channelled either to the JCC (during office hours) or the TTSH Contact Centre (after office hours) (Table 5).

Good analytics are also required to inform policy and workflow in the pandemic. The NCID Data Operations Team, previously known as the Data and Information Sense-making Team, continued to support the COVID-19 outbreak by making meaningful and evidence-based analyses to address the operational needs and queries from various internal and external stakeholders. With three additional FTEs on board since June 2020, the NCID Data Operations Team streamlined the data-extraction process and integrated additional data sets from multiple operations stakeholders to establish a comprehensive operational database. The team works closely with relevant stakeholders such as the National Public Health and Epidemiology Unit (NPHEU) and NCID IT team, and the Department of Clinical Epidemiology, TTSH. A COVID-19 data repository is being planned to archive the operational details and lessons learnt from the COVID-19 pandemic.

Ramping Up

With the increasing operations loads, the NOCC started full manning on 28 January, with augmented manpower garnered from various NCID departments. The requirements for manpower were pre-planned and deployed to commensurate with the scale of operations. As the outbreak situation evolved, the NOCC's scope also expanded to include managing foreign workers, transfers to Swab Isolation Facilities (SIF), etc. With the dynamic situation, constant adjustments had to be done to the workflow to adapt to policy changes and enhancements. The NOCC also collaborated with external agencies for these new workflows. For instance, the NOCC worked with the MOH EPR and Ministry for Home Affairs (MHA) to establish the workflows for managing persons under custody during screening and inpatient care.

There were initial challenges in gathering manpower for staffing the NOCC. However, with strong support from NCID departments, the NOCC managed to garner sufficient manpower to run the Operations Command Centre for 24/7 operations. From 25 March, the NOCC collaborated with TTSH to take over the operations of the campus JCC. The JCC also was concurrently expanded to include facilitating direct admissions of suspect COVID-19 patients to the NCID and TTSH outbreak wards.

TTSH provided support with augmented manpower for the operations of the JCC to keep pace with the increasing loads and expanded scope of operations. The NCID Infectious Disease Research and Training Office (IDRTO) also contributed manpower who were instrumental in providing leadership and guidance to the JCC team. The function of JCC continued to evolve as the focus of the outbreak changed, to include the arrangement of same-day decant to CCF, admission of patients for serology testing, etc.

Some challenges for JCC include the knock-on effect from constant evolving policies in enhancing COVID-19 management or keeping pace with evolving situations. Manpower for the JCC had to be continually trained to enable effective operations coordination. Multiple sessions were needed for each change/enhancement in policy/workflow as augmented staff members were on rotating shifts to juggle COVID-19 duties and BAU works.

Operations loads were reduced but at a sustained pace during Phase 2, and TTSH and the NCID started returning to BAU on the background of COVID-19 operations. NOCC and JCC operations were integrated with reduced manpower that were deployed 24/7 to commensurate with operations loads. Additionally, temporary manpower was recruited to progressively backfill the augmented manpower being released for BAUs.

Overview of Healthcare Response in Singapore

Across Singapore, all public and private hospitals also ramped up their operations to manage COVD-19 patients. Community care and recovery facilities were also set up to receive COVID-19 patients at the latter/recovery stage of their illness. These included facilities at convention sites like the Singapore Expo Halls, Changi Exhibition Centre and Big Box, Tuas South recreation centre, private hospitals and community hospitals such as Mount Alvernia Hospital, Farrer Park Hospital, Bright Vision Hospital, Sengkang Community Hospital and Yishun Community Hospital, and chalets, for example, D'Resort. Innovative strategies such as a Telemedicine/Mobile Medication (TM/MM) service was also implemented with the Woodlands Health Campus (WHC) decanted to D'Resort. As of 30 June, a total of 5,733 patients have been decanted to CCFs from the NCID and TTSH inpatient wards and Short Stay Units (SSUs).

Therapeutics for COVID-19 in Singapore

COVID-19 Therapeutics workgroup

What appeared at the beginning of the outbreak to be a predominantly ARI/pneumonia gradually transformed into a seemingly systemic disease in certain at-risk patient populations. Extrapulmonary features, including cytokine release syndrome (CRS), a multi-system inflammatory syndrome in children with Kawasaki Disease-like features, to thromboembolic manifestations (acute coronary syndromes, cerebral infarcts, deep venous thrombosis, and pulmonary embolism), made this unlike another novel respiratory virus (Lai et al., 2020). The infected populations also changed during the course of the pandemic: from overseas travellers and returning Singaporeans to pockets of seniors who had either been involved in social and religious interactions in clubs and churches or were residents in nursing homes, to the large migrant worker population living in local dormitories.

An NCID COVID-19 Therapeutics Workgroup comprising of infectious diseases physicians, haematologists, rheumatologists, pharmacists, virologists, and representatives from the Health Sciences Authority (HSA) and Chapter of Infectious Disease Physicians of the College of Physicians,

Singapore, was convened in March. Considering the lack of direct evidence initially for this newly identified infection, published systematic reviews, meta-analyses, cohort studies, case series, animal and *in-vitro* studies related to SARS and MERS were considered in initial versions of this guideline. Each recommendation was discussed and evaluated by the expert committee, screened for conflicts of interest, and then reviewed for strength and quality of the evidence. Subsequently, results of published COVID-19 specific randomised controlled trials were used to update the therapeutic guidance, e.g., the positive results for remdesivir and dexamethasone in patients requiring supplemental oxygen (NCID, 2020).

Where possible, patients with severe COVID-19 infection were offered access to clinical trials (e.g., remdesivir trials) before off-label therapies like intravenous anti-interleukin-6 inhibitors, e.g., tocilizumab, were offered, when best supportive care was ineffective and where hyperinflammation was suspected. Hydroxychloroquine, an antimalarial drug used in the treatment of rheumatic diseases like systemic lupus erythematosus (SLE), was used early on in the pandemic. It was touted for its antiviral and immunomodulatory effect but was subsequently found to be ineffective for treatment. Similarly, a regime comprising a 14-day course of ritonavir/lopinavir was also found to be ineffective (NCID, 2020).

Convalescent plasma is a time-honoured treatment modality for various infectious diseases. A Convalescent Plasma Programme was initiated jointly in May 2020 by the NCID, TTSH Haematology and the Centre for Transfusion Medicine, HSA, following the recovery of index patients who had volunteered to have their plasma taken and stored for use in patients in critical condition. As of 29 July, six patients have been treated in Singapore with this modality, all of whom survived COVID-19. However, further robust data is needed about the efficacy of this treatment from randomised controlled trials.

It also then became apparent that some young males in their 30s to 50s with no prothrombotic risk factors were developing acute ischaemic limb(s) from aortic thrombosis, deep venous thrombosis, and pulmonary embolism related to acute COVID-19 infection; this included a number of recovered patients. Although prophylactic or therapeutic anticoagulation was recommended for COVID-19 patients without contraindications, patients in Singapore were further risk-stratified, taking into consideration critical illness, immobility, and other bleeding risks, e.g., elderly patients with severe COVID-19 (NCID, 2020).

Pandemic Preparedness Planning

A campus-wide approach involving joint leadership and staff from medical, nursing, allied health, pharmacy, ancillary, support and operations is key to the successful management of any pandemic. The monthly meetings on clinical, operational workflows and training matters on the TTSH–IDOC (Infectious Disease Outbreak Clinical Group) platform, and the conduct of small and large MOH exercises, e.g., Exercise Sparrowhawk and Respiratory X table-top / command post exercises, were crucial in ensuring a successful and well-coordinated approach to the current COVID-19 pandemic.

Summary

COVID-19, unlike preceding pandemics, has presented unique challenges to healthcare systems worldwide. After Singapore's experience during the SARS outbreak in 2003, the preparatory work that ensued, including the establishment of the NCID, put Singapore in better stead to confront the current pandemic. Nevertheless, given the magnitude of the pandemic and also its protracted course, it is clear that a whole-of-healthcare response is needed, alongside the whole-of-government approach as led by the Multi-Ministry Taskforce for COVID-19. Systems need to adapt and move with evolving scenarios as new information becomes available in the pandemic.

References

Lai C-C, Ko W-C, Lee P-I et al. (2020) Extra-respiratory manifestations of COVID-19. Int J Antimicrob **56**(2):106024. https://doi.org/10.1016/j.ijantimicag.2020.106024

Lee PH, Vasoo S. (2020) COVID-19 — Where do we go from here? Singapore Med J. doi: 10.11622/smedj.2020060

NCID (2020). COVID-19 therapeutic workgroup. interim treatment guidelines for COVID-19, version 3. NCID, 6 July. https://www.ncid.sg/Health-Professionals/Diseases-and-Conditions/Pages/COVID-19.aspx. Accessed 29 July 2020.

8

COVID-19 Research — The Singapore Story

Ramona A. Gutierrez

Introduction

If past pandemics and epidemics have taught the world anything, it is that (i) a common characteristic for all pandemics is uncertainty, and (ii) science and timely conduct of research is key to addressing this uncertainty. Over the past years, several emerging infectious diseases have once and again challenged our preparedness and response models for pandemics. The most recent examples include SARS-CoV in 2002–03, H1N1 influenza in 2009, Ebola in West Africa (2014–16) and Democratic Republic of Congo (DRC) (2018–20), and Zika in Brazil in 2015. Science and research have progressively been recognised worldwide as key elements to consider as part of a country's integrated pandemic preparedness and response plans (Lurie *et al.*, 2013; Marston *et al.*, 2017; Walley & Davidson, 2010; Webb & Nichol, 2018). In Singapore, the development of a national pandemic preparedness research strategy was recommended by an Infectious Diseases Taskforce in 2015–16 (Ministry of Health, 2016a; 2016b). This enabled Singapore to build and leverage existing platforms and capabilities for a timely research response to the COVID-19 pandemic.

Enabling and Organising the COVID-19 Research Response in Singapore

Singapore's National COVID-19 Research Workgroup — A central coordination platform

On 23 January 2020, Singapore became one of the first Asian countries to detect COVID-19 cases outside of China (Ministry of Health, 2020). The day before, key representatives from several healthcare, research and public health institutions answered the National Centre for Infectious Diseases' (NCID) call to gather and start organising national research efforts on this novel coronavirus disease. At the time of writing (July 2020), this group, since known as the national COVID-19 Research Workgroup (RWG), has been meeting every week ever since that first discussion. Chaired by the NCID's Executive Director Professor Leo Yee Sin and her deputy, A/Prof David Lye, Director, Infectious Disease Research and Training Office (IDRTO), and advised by the Ministry of Health (MOH)'s Chief Health Scientist Prof. Tan Chorh Chuan, the Workgroup comprises representatives from the NCID, National Medical Research Council (NMRC), National Healthcare Group (NHG), National Public Health Laboratory (NPHL), Duke-NUS Medical School, A*STAR, DSO National Laboratories, National University of Singapore (NUS), National University Hospital (NUH) and Nanyang Technological University (NTU).

The COVID-19 RWG provided a regular platform for multi-disciplinary and multi-institutional exchanges on research conducted by key domain experts and stakeholders. In particular, it facilitated a continuous conversation between clinicians and researchers from specific research fields, such as virology, diagnostics, immunology, bioinformatics and modelling. This conversation was further guided and fuelled by views and insights from top representatives from public health, funding and ethics review entities, who, in turn, had a continuous awareness of the research issues and efforts at work, thereby enabling them to make informed decisions relative to their respective fields (e.g., funding) within expedited time-frames. Overall, the RWG platform allowed the convergence of multiple disciplines and the framing of all research questions and studies towards clear clinical and public health outcomes, aligned with the NCID's mission statement of "Protecting the people of Singapore from infectious diseases".

Preparedness for Pandemic Research Coordination

Singapore's coordinated research response through the spontaneous formation of the RWG did not, however, start from a blank page. Rather, it built upon prior pandemic research preparedness efforts.

Commissioned under the National Research Foundation (NRF)'s five-year Research, Innovation and Enterprise (RIE) 2020 Plan (National Research Foundation, 2016), the Health and Biomedical Sciences (HBMS)'s Infectious Diseases Taskforce (IDTF) released a report in 2016 (Ministry of Health, 2016a, 2016b) outlining a proposed national strategy to guide future efforts in infectious diseases research. Pandemic threats and pandemic preparedness research were among the several areas of focus identified by the IDTF. Following this recommendation, a Pandemic Preparedness Research Strategy (PPRS) was proposed, as well as the setting up of a dedicated office to execute the strategy and coordinate relevant research efforts at the national level. The Pandemic Preparedness Research Coordinating Office (PPRCO), nestled within the newly built NCID, was formed in March 2019. The Pandemic Preparedness Research Committee (PPRC), in charge of providing directions for strategy and guiding the PPRCO in its execution, was formed in September 2019 and held its first meeting in October 2019, just under three months before COVID-19 hit Singapore's shores. While the work of the newly formed PPRCO was still in early planning stages, with much of its focus being on preparedness and "peace-time" in late 2019, the existence of a dedicated office to coordinate national research efforts proved to be an essential asset during the pandemic that ensued in 2020.

PROTECT — A pre-approved research protocol as the backbone of national research efforts

A cornerstone of any research effort during a pandemic is clinical research response and early access to critical information and samples from affected patients to inform our understanding of the disease. A timely activation of clinical research response may make significant contribution to bending the pandemic curve (Webb & Nichol, 2018).

A key backbone of the research by the NCID and collaborators to better understand COVID-19 has been in PROTECT, a multi-centred prospective study to detect novel pathogens and characterise emerging infections. This pre-approved drawer protocol, led by the NCID and now covering all public hospitals in Singapore, was first developed in 2012. The purpose of PROTECT is to enable rapid access to invaluable patient samples for research purposes in the event of any infection caused by a novel infectious agent. The specific aims of the PROTECT study are to: (i) detect novel, previously undescribed pathogens, and characterise associated clinical features; (ii) prospectively characterise the transmission risk, clinical features, host and pathogen interaction and natural and treated history of emerging infectious disease pathogens; (iii) characterise at-risk population and population given vaccine or preventive treatment in terms of epidemiologic and laboratory features; and (iv) characterise the general/ background population in terms of epidemiologic and laboratory characteristics. In the context of COVID-19, the first PROTECT patient was recruited on 24 January, one day after Singapore reported its first confirmed COVID-19 case, illustrating Singapore's early preparedness efforts in promptly taking action in outbreak circumstances. On 3 March, the PROTECT study team was among the first few globally to publish a descriptive case series of COVID-19 patients, providing much-needed information on clinical features and course among patients diagnosed with SARS-CoV-2 infection early into the pandemic (Young *et al.*, 2020). The COVID-19 patients recruited under PROTECT have since been the core source of samples and information for all major national research efforts on understanding the disease and on outbreak control or management (Fig. 1).

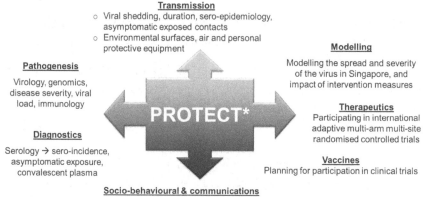

Transmission
○ Viral shedding, duration, sero-epidemiology, asymptomatic exposed contacts
○ Environmental surfaces, air and personal protective equipment

Modelling
Modelling the spread and severity of the virus in Singapore, and impact of intervention measures

Pathogenesis
Virology, genomics, disease severity, viral load, immunology

PROTECT*

Therapeutics
Participating in international adaptive multi-arm multi-site randomised controlled trials

Diagnostics
Serology → sero-incidence, asymptomatic exposure, convalescent plasma

Vaccines
Planning for participation in clinical trials

Socio-behavioural & communications
Public, healthcare workers, patients, quarantined exposed contacts, students, social media and fake news

* A Multi-centred Prospective Study to Detect Novel Pathogens and Characterize Emerging Infections. Pre-established outbreak drawer protocol led by NCID, developed in 2012

Figure 1. PROTECT — The pillar for critical research focus areas on COVID-19.

Funding urgent research

Funding has been a recurrent issue identified in Singapore (Ministry of Health, 2016a) and other nations (Lurie *et al.*, 2013; Webb & Nichol, 2018) in the timely conduct of crucial research during outbreaks. Fast disbursement of funds towards priority research areas requires strong political will, a sound understanding of the situation and immediate needs, as well as the assurance that precious monetary resources are indeed channelled towards capable entities that can effectively tackle research questions of most urgency. In Singapore, the RWG provided a platform where clinicians, researchers, NMRC funders and MOH policymakers sat at the same table. On this platform, the conversation was led by clinicians and researchers, with the NMRC as well as the MOH (represented by Chief Health Scientist Prof Tan Chorh Chuan) acting as advisors. As such, funders and policymakers were not the ones dictating the research directions. Rather, they were actively steering and advising a scientific discussion that was essentially contributed by clinicians and researchers while concurrently securing S$20 million for a special COVID-19 Research Fund that would be distributed in the first two of three tranches of funding (The Straits Times, 2020a).

Identifying and prioritising research areas

Several of Singapore's national research efforts have been fuelled by the weekly discussions of the RWG. Notably, from very early stages of the pandemic, the RWG helped identify and channel resources towards key priority areas of research. Those included research into disease pathogenesis and transmission, development of serology testing platforms, modelling of disease spread, and socio-behavioural aspects of the impact of COVID-19 on the population. The relevant teams were assembled for each of the themes identified, involving the relevant capabilities and expertise in each team, with some of the key parties (e.g., clinicians) involved in multiple teams. The Pandemic Preparedness Research Coordinating Office coordinated the submission of the proposals to the NMRC for expedited review. Within a few weeks, the proposals were approved (National Medical Research Council, 2020) and the researchers given the assurance that the priority work that they had been conducting since the start of the Singapore epidemic would be supported through these grants. While additional open grant calls subsequently followed, broadening the research scope to wider but somewhat less urgent issues, the expedited processing of the first tranche of funding ensured that priority efforts were already at work.

Adjusting ethics review processes to pandemic needs

With research priorities identified and funding released, another significant matter to enable the research is ethics approval. In "peace-time", the process of obtaining ethics approval, from writing the original protocol to undergoing ethics review by the Institutional Review Board (IRB) and obtaining final approval, typically takes anywhere from three to six months. In Singapore, two main entities are overseeing ethics considerations in research projects involving human subjects: the National Healthcare Group (NHG)'s Domain Specific Review Board (DSRB) and the Singhealth Central-ised Institutional Review Board (CIRB). By involving key leaders of both the NHG's and Singhealth's research arms from the start, the national COVID-19 RWG gave them continuous visibility over the fast-evolving research needs and context. By end-July 2020, the DSRB and CIRB had approved over 460 submissions (including new submissions and revisions), with a mean turnaround time of fewer than two weeks for new submissions, down to about a week for project amendments. Acknowledging the increasing number of COVID-19 projects and the decreasing bandwidth of the DSRB and CIRB, adjustments to their modus operandi were made to cope with additional COVID-19 submissions while allowing non-COVID-19 projects to proceed as well. These measures included the creation of additional domain boards to cope with the incoming volume.

Key Accomplishments and Outputs — Sharing with the Research and Healthcare Community

Monitoring of virus evolution globally through genomic surveillance

By the time COVID-19 hit the country, key research players in Singapore had already been hard at work building our understanding of the evolving situation in China. When the first genome sequence of the then-novel coronavirus 2019 (nCoV-19) was officially released by China on 12 January 2020 (World Health Organization, 2020b), the global research community, including Singapore, started putting their expertise and resources into investigating this novel agent. As a major technical partner of the Global Initiative on Sharing all Influenza Data (GISAID), a platform which promotes the international sharing of pandemic virus sequences, A*STAR's Bioinformatics Institute (BII), in particular, had a pivotal role in decrypting virus genomes and monitoring the virus evolution and its implications over time.

Research for diagnostics

In the early days, BII's work, in collaboration with A*STAR's Experimental Drug Development Centre (EDDC) and the Department of Laboratory Medicine (DLM) in TTSH, and with substantial support and guidance from the NCID's National Public Health Laboratory (NPHL) and A*STAR's Diagnostics Development (D × D) Hub, developed Fortitude Kit 2.0, a "ready-made" hospital laboratory diagnostic test kit (A*STAR, 2020). On 7 February 2020, less than a month after the release of the first nCoV-19 genomic sequence, Fortitude Kit 2.0 became the first kit to receive expedited provisional regulatory approval from Singapore's HSA for clinical use (Health Sciences Authority, 2020).

A "first-in-the-world" serology test

On 15 May 2020, the research team at the Duke-NUS Emerging Infectious Diseases programme announced the launch of a "first-in-the-world" SARS-CoV-2 serology test to detect neutralising antibodies without the need of a BSL-3 containment facility or specimen (The Straits Times, 2020b). This research was funded by the NMRC's first tranche of COVID-19 research funding (National Medical Research Council, 2020). The assay was developed in collaboration with GenScript, a biotechnology company, and A*STAR's DxD Hub and validated using samples of patients from the NCID's PROTECT study. The research team, however, did not wait till the official announcement of the kit's launch, or for the publication of the peer-reviewed manuscript in Nature Biotechnology in late July (Tan et al., 2020), to put the assay to use for public health purposes. Investigations of cases reported as early as from 29 January to 24 February used the Duke-NUS's serology assay to successfully link two people with COVID-19 from Wuhan, China, to three clusters of COVID-19 cases in Singapore (Yong *et al.*, 2020).

Contributing to international clinical trials for therapeutics

Early into the pandemic, the NCID joined the US National Institutes of Health (NIH)'s Adaptive COVID-19 Treatment Trial (ACTT), spanning 60 study sites in ten countries at the time of writing (August 2020) (National Institute of Allergy and Infectious Diseases, 2020). Singapore also joined Gilead Sciences' clinical trial platform, covering 183 study locations in 15 countries at the time of writing, and focusing on the evaluation of the highly promising drug Remdesivir (GS-5734TM) (Gilead Sciences, 2020). The prompt establishment of these collaborations was greatly facilitated through close exchanges with Singapore's HSA, which enabled expedited regulatory approval for the use of the drug. These collaborative trials placed Singapore at the forefront of the global search for an effective treatment for COVID-19, leading to much-awaited first publications on the trials' finding in late May 2020 (Beigel *et al.*, 2020; Goldman *et al.*, 2020). These early insights into the potential of remdesivir in managing clinical illness further informed treatment guidelines, both locally and for the international community's benefit (National Centre for Infectious Diseases, 2020b; Rochwerg *et al.*, 2020).

Ongoing Research — COVID-19, An Elusive Disease

Understanding host immune response and protection from SARS-CoV-2 infection

The race for safe and efficacious vaccines for SARS-CoV-2 is baffling all known vaccine development dogma and timelines, with close to 30 vaccine candidates in clinical trials (including six in Phase 3) within less than seven months into the pandemic (World Health Organization, 2020a). Yet, much remains to be elucidated on the host immune response to SARS-CoV-2 infection and mechanisms of protection from infection. Through PROTECT and thanks to well-established immunology monitoring platforms in A*STAR's Singapore Immunology Network (SIgN) and Duke-NUS Medical School, significant progress has been made to characterise and understand the immune response to COVID-19. While some of this work has been published (Le Bert et al., 2020; Poh et al., 2020), the characterisation of the neutralising antibody, T-cell and inflammatory responses is a key point of focus of Singapore's research efforts at the time of writing (August 2020).

Environmental transmission potential of SARS-CoV-2

In early July 2020, the World Health Organization (WHO) reportedly acknowledged "evidence emerging" of airborne spread of COVID-19 (Reuters, 2020), stirring global concern over the associated risk of transmission and the validity of the guidance issued earlier by the WHO on Infection Prevention and Control (IPC) practices. The NCID's IPC research team, in collaboration with DSO National Laboratories, was one of the first groups globally to closely examine and document environmental contamination by SARS-CoV-2 (Ong et al., 2020a; Ong et al., 2020b; Young et al., 2020). Recognising the need to further these efforts in order to answer key public health research questions on environmental transmission and intervention, several groups have since joined forces under Singapore's Chief Health Scientist Prof. Tan Chorh Chuan's helm to gather local capabilities and expertise. These groups include experts from the fields of building design and engineering, high-performance computing, metagenomics, and materials research and engineering. While the airborne transmission of SARS-CoV-2 is still at the centre of a global debate, evidence to ascertain this route of transmission is lacking, and through converging multiple disciplines towards this common goal, Singapore hopes to lead the way in generating evidence that directly supports interventions and policies.

The true extent of disease transmission in the community

While several efforts have been put into characterising SARS-CoV-2 transmission dynamics within the community, including in Singapore

(Kwok *et al.*, 2020; Wei *et al.*, 2020), the real basic reproductive number (R0), defined as the number of secondary cases infected by an index case in a susceptible population, has been eluding researchers and public health entities worldwide. As countries and economies attempt to gradually re-open (Dickens *et al.*, 2020), understanding the true extent of disease transmission so as to devise targeted intervention strategies has become a priority for many. In light of recent estimates of asymptomatic COVID-19 cases and associated "silent" disease transmission (Moghadas *et al.*, 2020), the NCID created a new discussion platform for closer exchanges between epidemiologists, clinicians, public health and modelling groups in Singapore to investigate these further. This will ensure again the conduct of research that is directly relevant to immediate public health needs, benefiting the community at large.

Socio-behavioural aspects of the COVID-19 pandemic

While much can be achieved through translating fundamental and clinical research findings to policy and intervention, the key to the success of intervention measures often lies in how the populations concerned receive, perceive and adopt these measures. This is why socio-behavioural studies were identified early on by the national COVID-19 RWG as one of the few priority research areas that needed immediate attention. The work conducted by the NCID, NUS and NTU researchers to better understand knowledge, risk perception, and behaviours towards the COVID-19 pandemic is providing insightful information that can help authorities communicate decisions and measures to the public (Lwin *et al.*, 2020; National Centre for Infectious Diseases, 2020a).

Monitoring vaccine developments worldwide

From a typical timeline of 10–15 years, the vaccine development timeline for COVID-19 is being reduced to 1–2 years. As of 13 August 2020, the WHO listed 138 candidate vaccines in preclinical evaluation and 29 candidate vaccines in clinical evaluation, including six in Phase 3 clinical trials

(World Health Organization, 2020a). Whether most of these vaccines will be successfully commercialised remains to be seen. In order to keep a close watch on the rapidly evolving vaccine development landscape worldwide, Singapore assembled a national panel advising on therapeutics and vaccines for Covid-19. This panel, involving several members of the RWG led by the NCID, has actively engaged leading vaccine groups and companies internationally (The Straits Times, 2020c). The objectives are for Singapore to participate in vaccine clinical trials, as well as to expedite regulatory review and approval for any successful vaccine.

Conclusion

The COVID-19 pandemic has had many lessons for the research community. It has unveiled our strengths, collaborative potential, resilience and ability to re-invent the way we think and operate. It has shown us the collective will to work together towards a common good, gathering clinicians, virologists, immunologists, public health officers, epidemiologists, bioinformaticians, policymakers, social scientists, funders, and several others, and converging forces towards understanding the disease and mitigating its impact on the community, together. It has demonstrated the value of having a continuous open research conversation among all parties to enable and accelerate research of immediate urgency, with several of these efforts translating into peer-reviewed publications for the global community to benefit from. The COVID-19 pandemic has unveiled our vulnerabilities to pandemics; the research scene in Singapore and beyond still has much to do to elucidate SARS-CoV-2. Learning crucial lessons from this pandemic shall allow us to rise from this challenge with stronger pandemic preparedness research programmes to enhance our response to future infectious diseases threats.

Note: this chapter was completed in August 2020. While the information gathered within was accurate as of August 2020, the COVID-19 research landscape has since evolved, both in Singapore and globally. In particular, the rapid development and deployment of COVID-19 vaccines, as well as the emergence of several Variants of Concern in late 2020, have influenced research priorities worldwide. As research directions keep adjusting as the pandemic evolves, further lessons will be learned, and hopefully inform and shape future pandemic preparedness research strategies.

References

A*STAR. (2020) Fighting COVID-19 with Fortitude. A*STAR HQ corporate web-site, 25 March. https://www.a-star.edu.sg/News-and-Events/a-star-news/news/covid-19/fighting-covid-19-with-fortitude

Beigel JH, Tomashek KM, Dodd LE *et al.* (2020) Remdesivir for the treatment of Covid-19 — Preliminary report. *New Eng J Med* **383**:1813–1826. https://doi.org/10.1056/NEJMoa2007764

Dickens BL, Koo JR, Lim JT *et al.* (2020) Modelling lockdown and exit strategies for COVID-19 in Singapore. Lancet Regional Health. https://doi.org/10.1016/j.lanwpc.2020.100004

Gilead Sciences. (2020) A phase 3 randomized study to evaluate the safety and antiviral activity of remdesivir (GS-5734TM) in participants with severe COVID-19. clinicaltrials.gov. https://clinicaltrials.gov/ct2/show/NCT04292899

Goldman JD, Lye DCB, Hui DS *et al.* (2020) Remdesivir for 5 or 10 days in patients with severe Covid-19. *New Eng J Med* **383**:1827–37. https://doi.org/10.1056/NEJMoa2015301

Health Sciences Authority, Singapore. (2020). The Health Sciences Authority of Singapore expedites approval of COVID-19 diagnostic tests as part of our national response to the public health emergency. https://www.hsa.gov.sg/docs/default-source/default-document-library/hsa-expedites-approval-of-covid-19-diagnostic-tests.pdf

Kwok KO, Chan HHH, Huang Y *et al.* (2020) Inferring super-spreading from transmission clusters of COVID-19 in Hong Kong, Japan, and Singapore. *J Hosp Infect* **105**(4):682–85. https://doi.org/10.1016/j.jhin.2020.05.027

Le Bert N, Tan AT, Kunasegaran K *et al.* (2020). SARS-CoV-2-specific T cell immunity in cases of COVID-19 and SARS, and uninfected controls. *Nature* **584**: 457–462. https://doi.org/10.1038/s41586-020-2550-z

Lurie N, Manolio T, Patterson AP *et al.* (2013) Research as a part of public health emergency response. *New Eng J Med* **368**(13):1251–55. https://doi.org/10.1056/NEJMsb1209510

Lwin MO, Lu J, Sheldenkar A *et al.* (2020) Global sentiments surrounding the COVID-19 pandemic on Twitter: Analysis of Twitter trends. *JMIR Public Health and Surveillance* **6**(2):e19447. https://doi.org/10.2196/19447

Marston HD, Paules CI, Fauci AS. (2017) The critical role of biomedical research in pandemic preparedness. *JAMA* **318**(18):1757–8. https://doi.org/10.1001/jama.2017.15033

Ministry of Health. (2016a) Infectious disease taskforce report. https://www.nmrc.gov.sg/docs/default-source/about-us-library/idtf-summary-report.pdf?s-fvrsn=c1fc317d_2

Ministry of Health. (2016b) Infectious disease taskforce report — Executive summary. https://www.nmrc.gov.sg/docs/default-source/about-us-library/idtf-executive-summary.pdf?sfvrsn=4650971e_2

Ministry of Health. (2020) MOH | News highlights — Confirmed imported case of novel coronavirus infection in singapore; multi-ministry taskforce ramps up precautionary measures. Ministry of Health, Singapore, 23 January. https://www.moh.gov.sg/news-highlights/details/confirmed-imported-case-of-novel-coronavirus-infection-in-singapore-multi-ministry-taskforce-ramps-up-precautionary-measures

Moghadas SM, Fitzpatrick MC, Sah P *et al.* (2020) The implications of silent transmission for the control of COVID-19 outbreaks. *Proc Nat Acad Sci USA* **117**(30):17513–15. https://doi.org/10.1073/pnas.2008373117

National Centre for Infectious Diseases. (2020a) NCID, NUS and NTU Studies Highlight the Role of Socio-Behavioural Factors in Managing COVID-19 - National Centre for Infectious Diseases. https://www.ncid.sg/News-Events/News/Pages/NCID,-NUS-and-NTU-Studies-Highlight-the-Role-of-Socio-Behavioural-Factors-in-Managing-COVID-19-.aspx

National Centre for Infectious Diseases. (2020b) Interim treatment guidelines for COVID-19. National Centre for Infectious Diseases, Singapore, 6 July. https://www.ncid.sg/Documents/COVID-19%20Therapeutic%20Workgroup%20-%20Interim%20Treatment%20Guidelines%20for%20COVID-19%20v3%20(6%20July%202020)%20-%20FINAL%20(ed).pdf

National Institute of Allergy and Infectious Diseases. (2020) A multicenter, adaptive, randomized blinded controlled trial of the safety and efficacy of investigational therapeutics for the treatment of COVID-19 in hospitalized adults. National Institute of Allergy and Infectious Diseases. clinicaltrials.gov. https://clinicaltrials.gov/ct2/show/NCT04280705

National Medical Research Council. (2020) NMRC | COVID-19 Research Projects. National Medical Research Council, Singapore. https://www.nmrc.gov.sg/grants/awarded-projects/covid-19-research-projects

National Research Foundation. (2016) RIE2020 plan. National Research Foundation, Singapore. https://www.nrf.gov.sg/rie2020

Ong SWX, Tan YK, Chia PY *et al.* (2020a) Air, surface environmental, and personal protective equipment contamination by Severe Acute Respiratory Syndrome Coronavirus 2 (SARS-CoV-2) from a symptomatic patient. *JAMA* **323**(16):1610–12. https://doi.org/10.1001/jama.2020.3227

Ong SWX, Tan YK, Sutjipto S *et al.* (2020b) Absence of contamination of personal protective equipment (PPE) by Severe Acute Respiratory Syndrome Coronavirus 2 (SARS-CoV-2). *Infect Control Hosp Epidemiol* 1–6. https://doi.org/10.1017/ice.2020.91

Poh CM, Carissimo G, Wang B *et al.* (2020) Two linear epitopes on the SARS-CoV-2 spike protein that elicit neutralising antibodies in COVID-19 patients. *Nat Commun* **11**(1):2806. https://doi.org/10.1038/s41467-020-16638-2

Reuters. (2020) WHO acknowledges "evidence emerging" of airborne spread of COVID-19. Reuters, 8 July. https://www.reuters.com/article/us-health-coronavirus-who-airborne-idUSKBN2482AU

Rochwerg B, Agarwal A, Zeng L *et al.* (2020). Remdesivir for severe covid-19: A clinical practice guideline. *BMJ* **370**:m2924. https://doi.org/10.1136/bmj.m2924

Tan CW, Chia WN, Qin X *et al.* (2020). A SARS-CoV-2 surrogate virus neutralization test based on antibody-mediated blockage of ACE2–spike protein–protein interaction. *Nat Biotechnol* **38**:1073–78. https://doi.org/10.1038/s41587-020-0631-z

The Straits Times. (2020a) The role of MOH's chief health scientist amid the Covid-19 pandemic. The Straits Times, 30 April. https://www.straitstimes.com/singapore/the-role-of-mohs-chief-health-scientist-amid-the-covid-19-pandemic

The Straits Times. (2020b). Singapore develops new test that can swiftly detect if someone has had Covid-19. The Straits Times, 15 May. https://www.straitstimes.com/singapore/health/coronavirus-singapore-develops-new-test-that-can-swiftly-detect-if-someone-has-had

The Straits Times. (2020c) Singapore's search for a cure and vaccine for Covid-19. The Straits Times, 23 May. https://www.straitstimes.com/singapore/health/finding-a-cure-and-vaccine-for-covid-19

Walley T, Davidson P. (2010) Research funding in a pandemic. *Lancet* **375**(9720):1063–65. https://doi.org/10.1016/S0140-6736(10)60068-2

Webb SA, Nichol AD. (2018) Bending the pandemic curve: Improving decision-making with clinical research. *Cri Care Med* **46**(3):442–46. https://doi.org/10.1097/CCM.0000000000002912

Wei WE, Li Z, Chiew CJ *et al.* (2020) Presymptomatic transmission of SARS-CoV-2—Singapore, January 23–March 16, 2020. *Morb Mortal W Rep* **69**(14):411–15. https://doi.org/10.15585/mmwr.mm6914e1

World Health Organization. (2020a) Draft landscape of COVID-19 candidate vaccines. https://www.who.int/publications/m/item/draft-landscape-of-covid-19-candidate-vaccines

World Health Organization. (2020b). Novel coronavirus — China — Disease outbreak news. World Health Organization, 12 January. http://www.who.int/csr/don/12-january-2020-novel-coronavirus-china/en/

Yong SEF, Anderson DE, Wei WE *et al.* (2020) Connecting clusters of COVID-19: An epidemiological and serological investigation. *Lancet Infect Dis* **20**: 809–15. https://doi.org/10.1016/S1473-3099(20)30273-5

Young BE, Ong SWX, Kalimuddin S *et al.* (2020). Epidemiologic features and clinical course of patients infected with SARS-CoV-2 in Singapore. *JAMA* **323**(15):1488–94. https://doi.org/10.1001/jama.2020.3204

9 Community Engagement and Response to COVID-19

Steven PL Ooi[1]

Introduction

Community engagement involves working in partnership with groups of people affiliated by special interests or similar situations to address threats to health and well-being. In 2020, Singapore took a turn for the worse when facing a surge of COVID-19 cases, it had to undertake massive operations to limit community spread (Wilder-Smith et al., 2020; Wee et al., 2020). Restrictive measures, known as Circuit Breaker (CB), were introduced from 7 April to 4 May and had to be extended until 1 June. The authorities ceased all mass gatherings and non-essential activities to break the chain of transmission, albeit with economic and financial consequences. When the CB ended, it was not possible to return to the community's pre-COVID-19 situation. The outbreak has significantly affected everyone in terms of health, work, and social interactions. In this chapter, we share our experience with community engagement and response to COVID-19, from the city-state's wake-up call and crisis management in the year 2020, to gearing up for the new reality.

Waking Up To Pandemic Preparedness

What is it like to be on our community frontlines against the virus? No one can be certain what will happen in the next one to two years until an effica-

[1] Senior Consultant, Infectious Disease Research and Training Office, National Centre for Infectious Diseases, and Associate Professor, Saw Swee Hock School of Public Health, National University of Singapore

cious control system becomes commonplace. The next wave may be even larger than the previous ones if we let our guard down. In the meantime, we are to prepare for the worst while hoping for the best. Throughout this time, we have caught glimpses of a future normal.

Disease control requires community cooperation

Pandemic preparedness institutionalises contact tracing as an investigative process of containment involving comprehensive case activity mapping, identification of persons who have come into contact with each case, and classifying them by close, casual or transient contact for appropriate public health actions (Fig. 1). Tracing the close contacts, testing them for infection, treating the infected and tracing their contacts, in turn, all aim to identify sources of infection in the community and interrupt ongoing transmission (Ng *et al.*, 2020; Tan *et al.*, 2020).

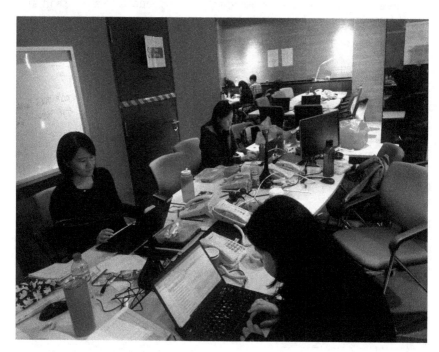

Figure 1. Community contact tracing is a cornerstone of COVID-19 control in a daily race against time to break the chain of transmission.

On 19 January 2020, a cluster was introduced by two pre-symptomatic Chinese nationals from Wuhan to six local congregants at the Life Church Missions, where they shared some activities. Elsewhere, between 29 January and 9 February, a symptomatic church worker at Grace Assembly of God inadvertently infected nine congregants and seven staff. The connection came only after a careful investigation found three persons to be critical links between the two churches through a private family event (Pung et al., 2020; Yong et al., 2020). Another cluster began on 15 February among members of a Hokkien singing group, triggered by a Chinese New Year dinner function held at SAFRA Jurong where one member who was symptomatic but afebrile had cleared temperature screening. Transmission propagated until 16 March as many continued to attend singing classes despite mild illnesses. In total, there were 48 cases comprising two teachers, 29 students, ten household contacts, and seven social contacts.

These clusters brought about more health checks and temperature screening at work and social places. Contact tracing provided these learning points for infection control:

- Stay home if sick (even if symptoms are mild)
- Avoid large gatherings over a prolonged period of time (of half an hour)
- Practice safe distancing (at least 1 m) at work and other places
- Reduce or avoid communal singing wherever possible
- Do away with or regularly clean shared items as common touchpoints
- Ensure common meals are individually served or packed
- Provide options for religious services online via digital means
- Promote work from home as the default practice

Consequently, public places and organised events routinely denied entry to symptomatic persons, and a registration system at the entrance was implemented for contact tracing purposes. Preschools, educational institutions, and eldercare services also operated under restrictive practices and curbs on visitors. Working from home, split teams, streaming services, online shopping, and food delivery soared.

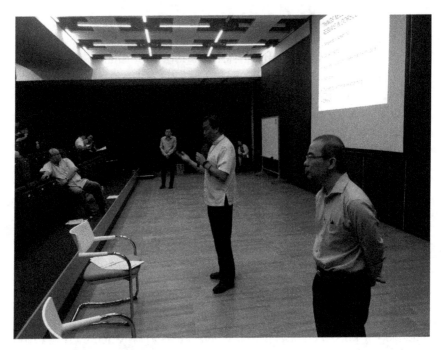

Figure 2.   The Catholic Archdiocese of Singapore convenes a presbyterium on 23 February for priests to discuss COVID-19 with medical guild doctors.

Preparing the ground for community cases

The identification of exposures at churches prompted religious and community leaders to critically review their existing practices in order to mitigate risks (Fig. 2). They were aided by the government providing public health advisories and holding dialogue across churches, mosques and temples. The media also did their part by drawing attention to messages from religious leaders on public concerns and the need to change certain practices in religious gatherings, which enabled members of the faithful to consider alternatives for worship and make bold decisions. This included the deferment of the annual Muslim haj pilgrimage.

Family physicians were among the first to be engaged in frontline response to the COVID-19 outbreak. On 14 February 2020, the Ministry of Health announced the re-activation of the country's Public Health Preparedness Clinics, which had been established after the 2003 SARS outbreak, and had seen service through the 2009 influenza pandemic and other emergencies. These clinicians and staff undergo periodic training to stay up-to-date with emergency outbreak protocols and serve as the first point of contact for patients with respiratory symptoms. The clinics enabled proper triage of cases, to offload case management from hospitals and reduce potential hospital-acquired infections.

At the same time, our National Centre for Infectious Diseases (NCID) and Saw Swee Hock School of Public Health linked up with community groups and the media to address concerns about outbreak response and risk communication. Independently, volunteers from the community stepped up to offer their services as safe distancing ambassadors. Retired healthcare professionals — many with the requisite skills and experience — also returned to work because they cared. Other members of the public continued to come forward to innovate, and support as best they can.

Grappling with Insecurity and Vulnerability

Urban health security entails efforts to minimise the impact of acute public health events that endanger the collective health of people in the community. Being a compact city-state with a high population density and dependent on global connectivity for our lifeblood, we have to accept the world as it is with many hard truths (Legido-Quigley et al., 2020). Part of this is acknowledging our insecurity and dealing with vulnerability.

Addressing signs of insecurity

In the early days of the outbreak, a crisis of public confidence took place, which moved faster than the crisis of public health. Masks, hand sanitisers and disinfectants were the first to fly off the shelves. Even in our traditionally stoic society, a breach in psychological defence was evident when many took to hoarding food and household items once Singapore moved to DORSCON Orange on 7 February. The authorities were quick to provide timely updates and dispel rumours. But people had different ways to judge the impact for themselves, with some even contemplating the "what-if" future state such as DORSCON Red. Their expectations and beliefs honed from prior experience and observation of other countries gave rise to panic buying and insecurity (Wei et al., 2020).

Insecurity amidst uncertainty is to be expected. Infodemics (excessive amounts of information) made their rounds in chat groups, stoking public anxiety, doubt and fear. Unfounded fears of infection even prompted members of the public to shun healthcare workers, and landlords to evict tenants who had worked in China. While social media is useful, it also means that information might be overstated because bad news spreads faster than good news. Moreover, there are built-in algorithms that prioritise sites similar to those often visited, compounding biases in line with previous viewpoints and worsening their adverse impact. Through hard-earned lessons correcting misinformation, systems were strengthened.

Community clusters, which arose sporadically, provided opportunities for us to derive valuable information, not just about the disease threat, but also about ourselves. Beyond the outbreak, one long-lasting positive effect took the form of a crash course on good personal habits and environmental hygiene. Community clubs, restaurants, supermarkets, shopping malls, wet markets, hawker centres, and public transport rigorously improved on cleanliness and waste management practices. The *SG Clean* campaign, together with apps such as *TraceTogether* and *SafeEntry*, helped to nudge the public on proper practices and responsible behaviour (Figs. 3 and 4).

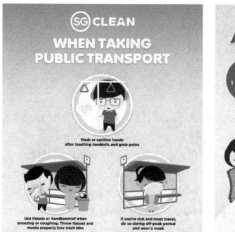
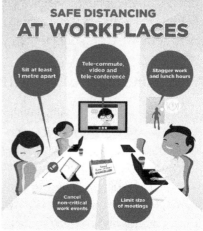

Figure 3. Examples of precautionary posters that promote community participation in disease prevention and control, released on 26 March.

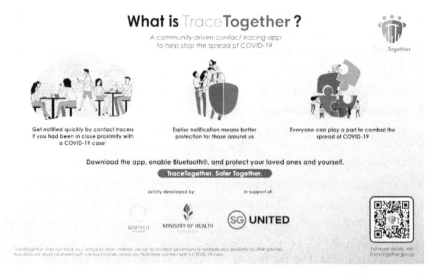

Figure 4. Advertising *TraceTogether* as a mobile application to promote community participation in contact tracing, launched on 20 March.

Managing vulnerability with migrant workers

Between 14 March and 26 April 2020, a defining moment came when 129 cases were traced to Mustafa Centre, a popular supermarket and shopping mall for tourists, migrant workers, and locals. In an analysis of the first 99 cases, 60 were staff, 18 were household or social contacts of staff, and 21 were visitors. The earliest cases included two staff members who had imported infection. One returned to work while symptomatic, while the other developed symptoms at work. Visitors had also gone to Mustafa while ill, and transmission spread via fomites at common touchpoints for customers. Temperature screening did not work since many cases reported no symptoms, and transmission likely propagated during staff breaks at common rest areas without safe distancing.

The virus took further advantage of migrant workers staying in packed dormitories and disseminated quickly into construction sites, workplaces and the community. Mega-clusters that developed highlighted our dependency on migrant workers and provided learning points in disease control:

- Temperature screening, though important, is not a fail-safe measure; cases with no/mild symptoms could be afebrile (Ho *et al.*, 2020)
- Safe distancing has to be reinforced at all events and shopping places
- Public-facing shops should introduce staggered shopping and regular cleaning of customer touch points (trolleys, baskets, ATM keypads)
- Loitering and aimless inter-mingling should be discouraged in public places
- Masks should be worn in public, and good hand hygiene practiced
- Workplaces should practice team segregation strictly
- Large-scale social events have to be postponed amid an outbreak

Our most significant lesson became the importance of personal responsibility. Transmission continued because people did not practice safe management. The truth about contagion is that we are scared to get it but less afraid to give it to others. Our community, and employers, must set the culture with responsible practices (for example, washing hands regularly with soap, avoiding crowded places, and monitoring our health closely) and show consideration for others (if feeling unwell, one should see a doctor or stay at home, observe respiratory etiquette, and dispose of soiled tissues in the rubbish bin). In the age of COVID-19, is it still tolerable that people leave behind discarded masks, used plastic water bottles and soiled tissues?

Future-Readying Our Community in Baby Steps

Singapore's CB managed to flatten the epidemic curve, but also much of the economy. Businesses are gradually reopening, mask-wearing and safe distancing have become common practices, but mass gatherings are still discouraged. While we struggle to chart a new path amidst COVID-19 fatigue, expenses and unemployment, community engagement is slowly building consensus on what constitutes acceptable risk (Park *et al.*, 2020).

Changing attitudes toward risk and routine

There are risks that affect multitudes without upsetting many, and there are risks that upset multitudes without affecting many. Gather together all the reasons people get upset and label them, collectively, the outrage factor. What the public perceives as risk is impact, which is the true risk plus the outrage factor (Moss *et al.*, 2016). Typically, the outrage factor is high when a new disease is unfamiliar, carries inconveniences, affects the pocket, and actions are not within personal control. Coming to the common ground requires a number of steps.

Firstly, people must expect to be impacted because we live in a susceptible environment. We remain porous because our borders cannot remain shut. As a major trade and travel hub with high people traffic, periodic re-introductions of the virus are inevitable. Travel will also encounter restrictions (Chinazzi *et al.*, 2020; Wells *et al.*, 2020). We will continue to see clusters arising from imported or locally acquired cases, usually by asymptomatic persons who may be unaware of their infection.

Secondly, the community must understand the difference between impactful inconveniences, such as panic buying, and true risk which guides public health actions. Risk is measured as the probability of getting infected and dying from exposure to the virus. Hence, through measures that reduce exposure, experts have calibrated a risk-based approach to health protection. Overcoming COVID-19 requires community support of these measures which can be personally intrusive (Fischbacher *et al.*, 2001).

Finally, we must adapt to the public impact by being less emotive (outraged) and by changing our daily routines in ways that reduce the stress of future disruptions. Supply chains are already disrupted, so we have to be judicious in our use of limited resources (Queiroz *et al.*, 2020; Guan *et al.*, 2020). Inconveniences are inevitable, so we must be patient instead of complaining. The outrage factor is not a distortion in the public's perception; it is an intrinsic part of having to deal with the impact.

Exercising consideration for at-risk groups

Mutual support becomes crucial in building our common defence against COVID-19. We must behave as though everyone around us is infectious and also assume that we are harbouring the virus so as not to pass it to others. We struggle with different emotions across different generations, and there are always conflicts of interest between personal liberties and the community good. Elders and the immunosuppressed may be pre-occupied with fear for their lives, while younger persons resent the loss of their economic and financial well-being. Our common purpose has already been tested in a spate of clusters, which occurred among seniors with limited mobility in residential care settings.

The first two clusters, one at Lee Ah Mooi Old Age Home affecting 14 residents (including two deaths), two staff and a household contact, and another at Acacia Welfare Home with 15 residents and two staff, ignited on 20 March and 11 April 2020, respectively. The virus was introduced from the community probably by asymptomatic workers, and this finding highlighted the need to pay attention to all homes that require regular contact between the elderly residents and attending staff. Rapid inter-sectoral response led to active surveillance at all nursing and welfare homes, heightened infection control, and public education to keep our vulnerable groups safe (Figs. 5 and 6).

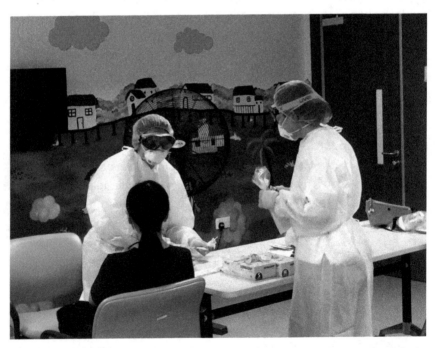

Figure 5. Screening of staff and residents at a nursing home on 13 April in response to the diagnosis of COVID-19 in one resident.

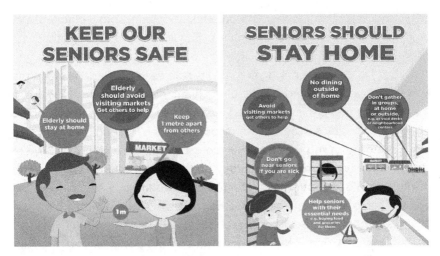

Figure 6. Senior-centric messages on prevention and control to help protect the vulnerable, released on 2 April (left) and 14 April (right).

What does the future hold? We rely on technological quick fixes to our problems although our weakest link is often a lack of consideration for others. A careless attitude erodes trust and builds suspicions. In an age of social capital deficit, the trust that our community places on someone who exercises personal responsibility must not be taken for granted. We should appreciate that relationships are built upon integrity and trust and that an effective whole-of-society approach requires these caring connections. As the national crisis unfolds on two fronts — public health and public confidence — we see a golden learning opportunity for us all to get this right.

Gearing Up Social Capital for the New Reality

The community-based response has become a vital asset in our fight against COVID-19. Our resourcefulness and country's size work in our favour — many challenges are much more manageable in scale here than they would be in other countries. As our community seeks the new normal in a post-circuit breaker world, we will make mistakes, but we must continue to innovate solutions. We learn even as we are already sailing and give leeway to discard what does not work without entering into a blame game. Our pluralistic society is a strength here, for we can do much together with decades of persistent nation building in our blood.

Our NCID is undertaking community studies to better understand the knowledge, attitudes and practices prevalent in our population, including views on government implemented measures such as MCs and stay-home notices. In an early survey, 30% of respondents felt discouraged from seeing a doctor, knowing that they may be issued a five-day MC and have to stay at home for the period until they receive a negative COVID-19 swab result. Post-CB, adoption of protective behaviours such as handwashing and the use of masks showed good compliance, and there is behavioural change in people to avoid crowded places.

Community engagement has shown up both obstacles and opportunities that lie ahead in reducing the impact of acute events that endanger us all. Social habits are steadily changing as stakeholders come around to the new reality. The community is leveraging not just on government but also on business, communal and people-to-people ties to bridge existing gaps. There have arisen sources to seek advice from, including credible non-government ones capable of dealing with critical feedback and public confidence. Community resilience is built on a network of trust and relationship. We must strengthen community bonds, for our future will be one of socially responsible choices.

The efficient systems that have served us well in the past were never built for care; it is individuals who care. Social responsibility is when, for the sake of others, we assess our necessity of travel or close contact, and if faced with a quarantine order or stay-home notice, we play our part through strict compliance. Many healthcare, frontline and public health workers have already borne sacrifices and inconveniences to help keep the rest of us safe (Htun et al., 2020). What these strenuous efforts are achieving is to buy us precious time to prepare for our new normal that invests in social capital. We have choices to make a difference for the future.

Social capital is strengthened by our concern for and openness to other views. We must remember that safe distancing is about physical and not social distancing. Bottom-up initiatives from the community are proving vital to Team Singapore. Acts of kindness when people cooperated to give unused masks and hand sanitisers to others or cheered on frontline workers with food and messages of love and care nourished hearts with a warm glow of togetherness. Our spirits are lifted by community stories of selflessness. A groundswell of goodwill occurs when people are motivated to rally for a greater cause to promote health security for all.

We see chances for us to improve our social capital with renewed norms of self-reliance, solidarity and cooperation — how to protect one another and make the best of every situation. The verdict on this outbreak is not out yet. Whether COVID-19 keeps mutating or becomes endemic, our wellbeing depends not so much on the disease but our collective resilience and response. In this way, we can enjoy life even as we make adjustments for the greater good. Indeed, we are preparing for a flexible future together where Singapore, faced periodically with emerging infections, can respond effectively.

Conclusion

Through community engagement, religious groups, businesses, social enterprises, nursing homes, shelters, and welfare and private organisations have worked with the public health and other authorities to gain insights and confront the new reality of COVID-19. Many opportunities exist to explore how we can cope better in this pandemic age. Engagement helps to mobilise resources and influence systems, strengthen relationships among partners, and serve as catalysts for new policies and practices. It is a powerful vehicle for bringing about improvements to all. We must be adaptable to safeguard health together in a brave new world.

References

Chinazzi M, Davis JT, Ajelli M *et al*. (2020) The effect of travel restrictions on the spread of the 2019 novel coronavirus (COVID-19) outbreak. *Science* **368**(6489):395–400.

Fischbacher U, Gächter S, Fehr E. (2001) Are people conditionally cooperative? Evidence from a public goods experiment. *Econ Lett* **71**:397–404.

Guan D, Wang D, Hallegatte S *et al*. (2020) Global supply-chain effects of COVID-19 control measures. *Nat Hum Behav* **4**:577–87.

Ho CS, Chee CY, Ho RC. (2020) Mental health strategies to combat the psychological impact of COVID-19 beyond paranoia and panic. *Ann Acad Med Singapore* **49**(3):155–60.

Htun HL, Lim DW, Kyaw WM *et al.* (2020) Responding to the COVID-19 outbreak in Singapore: Staff protection and staff temperature and sickness surveillance systems. *Clin Infect Dis*. doi: 10.1093/cid/ciaa468

Legido-Quigley H, Asgari N, Teo YY *et al.* (2020) Are high-performing health systems resilient against the COVID-19 epidemic? *Lancet* **395**(10227): 848–50.

Moss R, Hickson RI, McVernon J *et al.* (2016) Model-informed risk assessment and decision making for an emerging infectious disease in the Asia-Pacific Region. *PLoS Negl Trop Dis* **10**:e0005018.

Ng Y, Li Z, Chua YX, Chaw WL *et al.* (2020) Evaluation of the effectiveness of surveillance and containment measures for the first 100 patients with COVID-19 in Singapore — January 2–February 29, 2020. *Morb Mortal W Rep* **69**(11):307–11.

Park M, Cook AR, Lim JT *et al.* (2020) A systematic review of COVID-19 epidemiology based on current evidence. *J Clin Med* **9**(4):E967. doi: 10.3390/jcm9040967

Pung R, Chiew CJ, Young BE *et al.* (2020) Investigation of three clusters of COVID-19 in Singapore: Implications for surveillance and response measures. *Lancet* **395**(10229):1039–46.

Queiroz MM, Ivanov D, Dolgui A *et al.* (2020) Impacts of epidemic outbreaks on supply chains: Mapping a research agenda amid the COVID-19 pandemic through a structured literature review. *Ann Oper Res* 1–38.

Tan SS, Yan B, Saw S, Lee CK *et al.* (2020) Practical laboratory considerations amidst the COVID-19 outbreak: Early experience from Singapore. *J Clin Pathol*. doi:10.1136/jclinpath-2020-206563

Wee LE, Hsieh JYC, Puah GC *et al.* (2020) Respiratory surveillance wards as a strategy to reduce nosocomial transmission of COVID-19 through early detection: The experience of a tertiary hospital in Singapore. *Infect Control Hosp Epidemiol* **8**:1–16.

Wei WE, Li Z, Chiew CJ *et al.* (2020) Presymptomatic transmission of SARS-CoV-2 — Singapore. January 23–March 16, 2020. *Morb Mortal W Rep* **69**(14):411–15.

Wells CR, Sah P, Moghadas SM *et al.* (2020) Impact of international travel and border control measures on the global spread of the novel 2019 coronavirus outbreak. *Proc Nat Acad Sci USA* **117**:7504–09.

Wilder-Smith A, Chiew CJ, Lee VJ. (2020) Can we contain the COVID-19 outbreak with the same measures as for SARS? *Lancet Infect Dis* **20**(5): e102–07.

Yong SEF, Anderson DE, Wei WE *et al.* (2020) Connecting clusters of COVID-19: An epidemiological and serological investigation. *Lancet Infect Dis* **20**(7):809–15. doi: 10.1016/S1473-3099(20)30273-5

10 Maintaining Business-As-Usual for NCID Clinical and Public Health Functions During COVID-19 Pandemic

Christine Gao and Wong Chen Seong

Introduction

Harnessing the experience and lessons learnt from past pandemics like the 2003 Severe Acute Respiratory Syndrome (SARS) and 2009 Influenza A (H1N1) outbreaks, the National Centre for Infectious Diseases (NCID) was carefully conceptualised and purposefully built to enhance infectious disease outbreak management and public health preparedness for Singapore. Besides clinical services, the NCID houses six public health units,[1] each anchoring core areas in epidemiology, laboratory diagnostics, outbreak research and training, public health education and community engagement in key areas such as antimicrobial resistance, HIV and tuberculosis (TB).

Following its successful launch in September 2019, the NCID was prepared and poised to engage global, regional and local public health and infectious disease stakeholders and establish a foothold in Singapore's medical ecosystem. Within a short span of time, each of the six public health units under the NCID has fully anchored themselves in their domain areas

---

[1] The six public health units are National Public Health and Epidemiology Unit (NPHEU), National Public Health Laboratory (NPHL), Infectious Disease Research and Training Office (IDRTO), Antimicrobial Resistance Coordinating Office (AMRCO), National Public Health programme for HIV (NHIVP) and Singapore Tuberculosis Elimination Programme (STEP).

and executed their national mission to improve the health of the Singapore population and enhance Singapore's capability to respond effectively to infectious disease outbreaks.

Timeline for Singapore Transition From Disease Outbreak Response System Condition (DORSCON) Green to Yellow to Orange

The first cluster of severe pneumonia cases caused by a novel SARS-like virus in Wuhan, China, was reported to the World Health Organization (WHO) on 31 December 2019. Upon assessing its potential to spread beyond China, the NCID began preparations in developing diagnostic assays and outbreak management plans in anticipation of these novel SARS-like cases in Singapore. Together with Singapore's Ministry of Health (MOH), the NCID jointly developed the clinical guidance on the novel coronavirus, which would provide guidance to local medical practitioners on the management of suspect cases.

Within the NCID, key changes, such as the establishment of a special precaution area to screen suspect cases and the operationalisation of a dedicated ward for the admission of suspect cases, were implemented swiftly in early January. A special NCID Operational Command Centre (NOCC) was partially established to serve as the nerve centre to coordinate between multiple internal and external stakeholders to ensure inter-operability. The maintenance of these communication channels is crucial for the NCID to maintain oversight on the entire COVID-19 outbreak response and to increase efficiency for joint operations, especially for an evolving outbreak.

With increasing reports of novel coronavirus pneumonia cases detected in Wuhan and the subsequent exportation of cases to other cities and countries, the MOH raised the alert level from DORSCON Green to DORSCON Yellow on 21 January 2020. Three days later, the NCID confirmed its Singapore's first case of novel coronavirus infection from a tourist from Wuhan, the epicentre of the outbreak. In Singapore, despite border control, active screening, and rapid quarantine of close contacts, local cases without any links to previous cases or travel history to China were found. With the increasing number of local cases in Singapore, the

MOH raised the alert level from DORSCON Yellow to DORSCON Orange on 7 February, indicating that local transmission had taken place and there was a risk of community transmission.

As the disease spread across an increasing number of new cities and continents, the outbreak was officially declared a Public Health Emergency of International Concern (PHEIC) by the WHO on 30 January 2020. The WHO subsequently renamed the novel coronavirus as COVID-19 on 11 February and officially declared COVID-19 a pandemic on 11 March.

Impact of Coronavirus in Business-As-Usual in NCID

At the start of the pandemic, the NCID took advantage of the lead time in early January 2020 to review the business continuity plans (BCP) of all NCID clinical and public health programmes and make strategic plans in response to the evolving outbreak. One of the key initiatives of the NCID BCP was to split teams to ensure continuity of leadership and services. Each team was split into different locations, therefore video-conferencing was implemented to keep dispersed teams connected and aligned with the overall strategic approach.

The functions of the six public health units remained largely intact in the early phase of the outbreak, and selected staff were roped in from the public health units to assist in the operationalisation of critical response areas such as the NOCC and NCID screening centre prior to the augmented manpower support from Tan Tock Seng Hospital (TTSH). The majority of the six public health units' activities were ramped up to support COVID-19-related training, research, diagnostics and data analytics. Despite the shift of activities towards COVID-19 outbreak preparedness and management, HIV and TB remained key diseases of focus in the NCID and clinical care towards these patients, although altered, were not compromised.

As Singapore's first responder for novel infectious disease management, it was critical for the NCID to maintain sustainable manpower to deliver essential services throughout the entire operations. The NCID has a synergistic working relationship with TTSH. Campus level policies such as manpower and personal protection equipment policies were communicated and implemented throughout the Novena Health Campus since January 2020. The policies included the cancellation of pre-planned overseas and training leave to ensure that there was adequate manpower at the NCID with support from TTSH to manage the surge in cases locally. These policies were made ahead of the MOH's recommendations to all public healthcare institutions in Singapore. As such, staff were engaged continuously on the evolving policies to ensure they understood the policies and their concerns were addressed, especially on leave and overseas travel restrictions.

Apart from leave restrictions, all staff members on the Novena Health Campus area were required to adhere to the prevailing mask up policies, to report their temperature readings twice a day, and to seek medical attention when feeling unwell. The transition from DORSCON Yellow to DORSCON Orange also saw a significant reduction of face-to-face inter-actions and an increased proportion of work from home arrangements and teleconferences. In DORSCON Orange, the increased cross-institutions movement restrictions affected the traditional outreach and activities such as anti-microbial resistance education and audits on healthcare institutions. The manpower to run these activities was rapidly redeployed to assist in other growing COVID-19 related areas such as data management, epide-miological contact investigations and research.

This is only possible as core public health streams are amalgamated under one roof in the NCID and this enhances the NCID's ability to nimbly redeploy internal manpower to enhance inter-operability for COVID-19 response to support core and critical functions such as NCID clinical ser-vices, epidemiology and operations.

Maintaining Business-As-Usual for NCID Clinical Services

The Department of Infectious Diseases (ID) provides a wide variety of clinical services under the auspices of both the NCID and Division of Medicine, TTSH, for both outpatient and inpatient care. The COVID-19 pandemic response necessitated a rapid and extensive adaptation of extant clinical services, as manpower and resources had to be channelled into the diag-nosis, isolation, management and surveillance of COVID-19 cases. This strategy was implemented with the following guiding principles:

1. Ensuring the safety of patients and staff

In accordance with national policies to reduce the risk of transmission of COVID-19 at healthcare facilities, measures were introduced to reduce human traffic at the NCID, including deferring or cancelling patient appointments, cessation of visitor privileges, and reducing the number of on-site staff. Safe distancing measures in various clinical and public settings within NCID were also strictly enforced.

2. Ensuring that patient care was not compromised

The clinical services provided within the NCID are unique and essential for the health and well-being of its patients. This includes HIV continuity care, general Infectious Diseases (ID), travel health and vaccinations, Outpatient Parenteral Antibiotic Therapy (OPAT) and inter-departmental consultations. Despite the general scaling back of routine, "peace-time" services, it was of paramount importance that patient care was maintained through a rigorous process of triage and prioritisation to ensure timely and quality care.

3. Exploring the use of task-shifting and innovative solutions

With the limitations outlined above, a number of clinical services had to be adapted for the sake of safety and efficiency. These include the adoption of technological innovations (such as the use of telemedicine), task-shifting (such as the deployment of staff within departments and clinics to optimise manpower efficiency) and the employment of patient-centred services (such as ramping up of home delivery of chronic medications for patients).

Outpatient ID Services

HIV outpatient services

The NCID Clinical HIV Programme provides continuity care for more than 4,000 people living with HIV (PLHIV) and oversees the largest and most established HIV care centre in Singapore. During "peace-time" there are between 300 to 500 unique visits per week for HIV care at the Specialist Outpatient Clinic (SOC) J, which is the ID outpatient clinic in the NCID. These include visits for HIV continuity care, as well as walk-in consultations for acute illnesses, and visits to the HIV co-morbidity co-management clinics (HIV-Ophthalmology, HIV-Dermatology, HIV-Endocrinology and HIV-Psychiatry). Patients may also attend non-clinical services such as specialist Pharmacist visits for drug adherence counselling, psychological support and counselling with their Medical Social Workers, and a suite of Nursing and Allied Health services, including routine vaccinations, dietetics and nutrition, and physical and occupational therapy.

This high patient volume, as well as the concern that PLHIV may be at increased risk of COVID-19 infection and/or severe disease due to HIV-associated immune suppression, meant that measures needed to be implemented to reduce patient footfall and minimise transmission to patients at SOC J. Moreover, as the number of suspect and confirmed COVID-19 patients increased over the months of the pandemic, as well as in tandem with contact tracing efforts, the need for ID expertise increased accordingly. This led to the need to divert clinical manpower from routine HIV care into outbreak response sectors. This is especially pertinent given that nearly all ID specialists within the NCID run their own HIV continuity clinics either weekly or twice weekly, and so this manpower diversion resulted in a need to significantly reduce the HIV patient caseload during the pandemic response.

Accordingly, SOC J instituted measures to scale down patient attendances for routine outpatient care by 50% to 70%, with non-essential visits deferred to a later date, which effectively prolonged the interval between patient reviews from the generally recommended six-month period. This necessitated a process of careful clinical triage to determine which patients were deemed suitable for deferred review, usually to a date several months later. The criteria for safe deferral included the following: durable viral suppression, no previous history of recurrent default on scheduled clinic appointments, and no opportunistic infections or other co-morbid conditions requiring expedient follow-up and care. Patients who did not meet these criteria were given appointments for clinic review, which took place at HIV clinics run by covering physicians with a reduced number of patient visits. Delaying appointments for newly diagnosed patients was avoided, as they required timely review and early initiation of antiretroviral therapy to ensure the best possible outcomes. The Clinical HIV Programme also oversees a number of co-morbidity co-management clinics, such as the HIV-Psychiatry, HIV-Endocrinology, HIV-Ophthalmology and HIV-Dermatology clinics, with the aim of comprehensively co-managing the complex needs of an ageing population of PLHIV with concomitant chronic medical illnesses. These clinics also had to be similarly managed to reduce the co-mingling and potential cross-infection of physicians from outbreak and non-outbreak sectors of the respective hospitals. Apart from patient consultations, other clinical services that also had to be scaled down or deferred, included nurse-led vaccination programmes, in-person drug-adherence counselling and comprehensive sexual health clinics. Finally, SOC J actively engaged patients to increase the uptake of home delivery of medications, to ensure that adherence to essential medications (especially antiretroviral therapy for HIV) was not interrupted despite the need to reduce physical clinic or pharmacy visits.

SOC J pioneered the use of video-consultation for PLHIV with stable HIV infection in 2017, offering patients an option of alternating conventional in-person visits with secure video calls with their primary HIV physicians, with the primary intention of saving them travelling and waiting time. This telemedicine platform has since been further broadened to include tele-drug adherence counselling and directly observed antiretroviral therapy in efforts to reduce barriers-to-care and improve patient outcomes. The COVID-19 pandemic response led to an accelerated expansion of video-consultation for PLHIV, as it allowed a higher volume of patients to be seen safely and efficiently, without the need for physical visits to the clinic.

With the gradual and progressive resumption of routine clinical and other services, it would be important to study the impact of COVID-19 outbreak on HIV care services and PLHIV, including its effect on the overall population-level HIV viral load, the incidence of HIV-associated opportunistic infections and other AIDS-defining conditions, as well as the control of other chronic medical conditions in PLHIV.

General ID Outpatient Services

General ID cases constitute approximately 30% of the usual patient load during "peace-time". These cases include patients referred for diagnosis and management of episodic acute ID conditions, such as dengue fever, malaria and other tropical infections, pyrexia of unknown origin, as well as follow-up for more subacute and chronic infections, such as TB and other mycobacterial infections, and chronic bone and joint infections. These patients are seen in SOC J, and any who require special precautions (such as airborne precautions for suspected TB or measles or contact precautions for zoster) are triaged for management in the purpose-built SPA within SOC J.

The COVID-19 pandemic in Singapore coincided with a surge in dengue cases in the community in the first seven months of 2020, with a concentration of dengue cases in central Singapore — the catchment area — of patients referred to the NCID for medical care. As such, a scale-down of general ID services during this time was not possible, and this resulted in a proportionate deployment of manpower and resources to the dengue outbreak. Other acute, subacute and chronic general ID cases were then subjected to the same process of prioritisation and triage as outlined above for HIV cases, and they continued to be seen at SOC J and the SPA. This serves as a good reminder that the national outbreak response plan for communicable diseases needs to take into account the possibility of outbreaks involving multiple pathogens.

The Travel Health and Vaccinations Clinic (THVC) and the Outpatient Parenteral Antibiotic Therapy (OPAT) clinic are two subspecialty clinics housed physically in TTSH, which provide clinical ID services. The THVC, which provides pre-travel health evaluations and vaccinations for travellers as well as post-travel screening and treatment for travel-related illnesses, scaled down its services during the COVID-19 outbreak response period. There was a cessation of walk-in consultations, and only visits by appointment were allowed. Given the concomitant travel restrictions during this time, demand for THVC services was accordingly much reduced. However, essential urgent services continued, specifically, urgent rabies post-exposure evaluation and management. The OPAT clinic plays an essential role in right-siting patients requiring parenteral antibiotics, essentially reducing the number of inpatients through the provision of intravenous therapy in the clinic or at home. As such, with the exception of the discontinuation of home OPAT visits by OPAT nurses, all other OPAT services continued during the COVID-19 pandemic response period.

Inpatient ID Services

Routine inpatient ID services include inpatient management of patients with HIV and general ID conditions, as well as the provision of inter-departmental consultations, blood culture advisory services, and antibiotic stewardship services.

During the initial COVID-19 pandemic response period, the NCID was dedicated to managing COVID-19 cases and the need to rapidly ramp up the inpatient bed capacity for the management of suspect and confirmed cases of COVID-19. As such, routine services were displaced and relocated to TTSH. In essence, the entire inpatient capacity of NCID was converted to manage COVID-19 cases. Accordingly, TB, HIV and general ID inpatient cases alike were transferred to TTSH and managed by the Internal Medicine teams, with input from ID physicians to ensure that there was continued speciality care for these patients, especially those with complications. A dedicated ID team was rostered to provide daily consults and input for these patients. As the number of suspect and confirmed COVID-19 patients declined with the evolution of the outbreak locally, there was a phased and gradual return of inpatient ID services.

Inter-departmental consultations and blood culture advisory services constitute an essential ID service to the hospital at large and were not interrupted during the pandemic response period. ID specialists were rostered to provide these subspecialty consults. However, inter-hospital ID consultation services ceased due to restrictions on the movement of healthcare professionals between institutions and were enforced to reduce the risk of transmission of COVID-19 within the healthcare ecosystem. This meant that routine ID consult coverage of KK Women's and Children's Hospital and Ang Mo Kio Community Hospital, which form part of the "peace-time" workload of NCID ID physicians, had to be converted to phone consultation during this period.

Summary

At the time of writing, Singapore has gone through a period of strict mobility restriction and is progressively relaxing restrictions. The daily number of new cases from local transmission had been maintained at a single digit for several weeks. Slightly more than 100 COVID-19 cases were being cared for in acute hospitals. The system is progressively returning to its pre-COVID-19 state while keeping a dedicated capacity and resources in readiness to mount immediate response should a surge occur. As highlighted in this chapter, the COVID-19 pandemic response resulted in significant disruptions to the day-to-day work of the NCID, specifically with regard to clinical services. However, concerted and directed efforts have been taken to ensure that patient care and safety are not compromised. The experience of having to respond quickly to a rapidly changing and dynamic pandemic situation has undoubtedly shaped the way that this young organisation as a whole will grow and adapt to being ready to meet future emerging infectious disease challenges head-on. The post-COVID-19 world is anticipated to bring significant changes to the way in which inpatient and outpatient healthcare are provided. For planning purposes, we will need to consider the concerns of patient crowding, staff safety, and the decentralisation of medical care so as to future-proof the healthcare system.

11 Public Health In Action Over At the Migrant Worker Dormitories

Clive Tan and Iain Tan

This was going to be a *Diamond Princess*… but on land. That was our first initial thought. What followed was a script that no one could have predicted, although my team and I tried very hard to. Armed with the knowledge of communicable disease epidemiology, years of experience in the medical field, experience with medical operations, and a strong desire of wanting to help, we plunged straight into this operation and became part of an epic that stretched beyond our imagination.

When we first arrived at the Headquarters of the Joint Task Force (Assurance) on 8 April 2020, it was a hive of activity. The Task Force had just been assembled and comprised public officers from the Ministry of Manpower (MOM), Ministry of Health (MOH), Singapore Armed Forces (SAF) and Singapore Police Force (SPF). [Having undergone training as a military medical officer, this felt like a War Room.] The officers came together to share whatever information they had for a collaborative and collective sense-making of the situation at hand, and to think of what needed to be done quickly as a priority to get the situation under control.

And that was how April 2020 went — sense-making and doing what we could to get the situation under control. But the virus had other plans. The spread within the dormitories appeared unfettered by our attempts to institute infection control and safe distancing measures. But the actions taken in April had, in fact, changed the trajectory of the epidemic curve but with a lag of one to two weeks due to the disease incubation period.

So that was the genesis of the Medical Intel team at Joint Task Force (A), also known as JTF(A), which took on various forms during the course of the operation. It remained a critical feature and capability of the medical and operations response to managing the disease transmission in the dormitories, and it was eventually folded in as a permanent feature of the MOM structure.

The Medical Intel team provided a daily monitoring report of the COVID-19 situation in the dormitories (Fig. 1) and was tasked to provide insights on matters that had a bearing on the epidemic trajectory.

To better illustrate how these "early days" were like, there was (1) a strong uptick in the epidemic curves across several dormitories and the typical plateaus associated with the late phase of epidemic curves were not seen yet, (2) national testing resources were limited, (3) efforts to implement public order and public health measures by the ground Forward Assurance and Response (FAST) Teams, and (4) concern about the medical care provision in for the dormitory residents.

ABOUT FAST TEAMS

Forward Assurance and Support Teams, or "FAST" teams, comprise officers from the Ministry of Manpower, Singapore Armed Forces and the Singapore Police Force. More than 170 FAST teams had been deployed. This included 43 teams stationed at all purpose-built dormitories, and 127 mobile FAST teams providing coverage to factory converted dormitories, construction temporary quarters and private residential premises. The FAST personnel look into all aspects of the workers' well-being, which was a top priority. This ranged from availability of food and maintenance of hygiene to facilitating their medical care and remittance needs.

https://www.gov.sg/article/pulling-together-fast-to-ensure-the-well-being-of-migrant-workers

---

I recall in April that the Medical Intel team had to advise on several topical issues:

(a) The best way to approximate the extent of the spread within the dormitories.

Purpose Build Dormitory

14-Apr	15-Apr	16-Apr	17-Apr	18-Apr	19-Apr	20-Apr	21-Apr	22-Apr	23-Apr	24-Apr	25-Apr	26-Apr	27-Apr	28-Apr	29-Apr	30-Apr
1394	807	2329	2809	3467	3826	5067	5779	6442	7197	7770	8185	8837	9184	9473	9835	10125
702	52	978	1128	1375	1506	2081	2283	2297	2320	2344	2350	2363	2374	2386	2409	2419
27	52	109	162	261	295	479	540	620	721	816	832	866	886	902	911	936
184	275	345	406	489	501	520	610	677	759	831	837	844	859	869	889	896
14	24	29	59	75	88	139	161	216	225	241	281	329	345	355	366	370
15	20	32	53	96	116	131	158	186	210	244	273	289	314	321	328	336
6	9	15	40	53	56	123	224	240	248	251	283	288	300	316	338	351
6	9	152	162	165	166	185	198	210	234	254	267	272	280	301	310	316
31	44	45	55	79	82	114	132	161	179	207	229	250	275	298	306	316
1	6	38	51	58	64	83	98	117	144	166	183	205	219	234	257	274
46	55	75	85	97	100	135	146	166	180	196	209	218	226	231	239	244
15	21	33	40	46	64	93	106	124	148	165	177	190	201	215	222	229
95	109	113	125	136	138	141	150	158	162	170	177	182	191	200	204	209
4	9	15	24	34	64	68	85	96	105	124	138	151	154	170	176	200
5	5	8	9	23	37	50	56	79	101	108	111	130	131	140	140	151
80	86	88	94	97	97	97	101	106	109	110	110	119	126	131	132	133
4	5	2	4	27	33	58	54	80	90	92	97	100	101	102	119	120
1	2	8	10	5	14	17	62	66	92	94	105	108	108	105	111	119
43	64	77	83	90	95	96	98	103	104	106	106	107	108	108	109	109
14	21	25	34	40	46	53	55	62	67	72	83	95	100	103	107	109
3	3	3	9	10	14	29	28	31	42	43	45	47	63	70	76	108
2	4	7	12	20	25	28	28	33	39	54	67	77	88	96	103	106
51	57	65	66	67	73	74	78	78	79	81	81	83	86	87	87	90
17	18	18	25	26	27	29	29	33	37	38	42	56	61	74	76	83
3	3	3	1	1	1	2	3	31	33	42	49	316	320	320	320	341
3			17	17	17	21	23	32	254	258	262	267	273	274	279	291
3	4	6	7	1	1	1	2	33	33	40	155	182	190	198	206	220
			5	16	23	26	35	55	83	153	155	161	182	188	199	205
1	4	5	5	8	10	78	78	108	112	113	117	123	133	144	152	159
3	2	3	6	6	6	31	31	79	92	98	100	100	101	101	111	112
3	14		14	17	17	17	21	31	62	81	81	82	91	92	95	98
11	14	14	16	17	17	17	21	23	28	29	29	37	40	41	46	60
11	11	12	12	14	16	19	20	20	22	23	27	29	31	31	31	33
4	5	5	5	5	5	6	6	9	11	12	13	14	15	16	20	21
	1			2	4	12	16	41	41	41	44	46	49	71	138	140
1	1	1	1	1	1	1	4	7	19	30	30	32	80	80	80	84
1			1	2	3	2	3	3	6	7	8	15	15	15	16	39
3	4	3	5	2	3	3	3	5	5	14	15	29	29	31	36	37
			1	1	6	6	6	19	19	19	19	20	20	23	25	26
1	1	1	1	1	1	3	4	5	5	12	13	14	15	16	16	16
		1		1	1	2	2		1	1	1	15	15	15	16	16
			1	1	1	2	2	2	2	2	2	2	2	2	2	2
0	0	0	0		1	2		2	0	1	0		2	1	1	1

Figure 1. Daily monitoring chart presented by the Medical Intel team, from 30 April 2020.

(b) Practicable public health interventions that could reduce and arrest the transmission of the disease.
(c) Using the data available, predict where the next outbreaks would occur and advise on timely pre-emptive interventions for these sites.

We were working at the frontiers of science and public health. New research and publications were emerging and the operational situation was evolving, the plans had to be steered in response to changes in the above. We had to be closely plugged into the medical operations to advise on the planned interventions and serve as a source of data and information.

It was an emotional rollercoaster, but we did not let it show. Our informational products and demeanour were always professional, but internally and behind closed doors, we did ponder aloud on whether we could have done more, thought further, worked harder, and slept lesser. Every time we discovered a new insight that could make a difference, there was a burst of excitement and a recharge of our batteries. Whenever we made the right call on which were the high-risk sites that could be undergoing an undetected outbreak, there was a sense of professional satisfaction and encouragement. But every time we got flanked and outsmarted by the virus or the realities of the difficult operating environment, we would feel deflated (although we would never admit it publicly) and had to reach into the deep recesses of our training to pick ourselves up again to get back into the daily battle rhythm.

Amidst Events Unfolding and Being Part of History

At the end of April (which was also the Circuit Breaker [CB] period), this was how the situation was like:

(a) The community cases were still high but starting to tail down (see the epidemic curve in Fig. 5).
(b) The number of cases coming from the dormitories was high and still on the rise.

(c) The hospitals were overloaded, and stable patients were decanted to community isolation facilities, with plans to repurpose general sites such as the Singapore Expo to become community isolation and care facilities.

While things appeared to have gotten worse in end-April, we were in a better place than in early April, in terms of better overall situational awareness, by having levers of control and intervention and putting in place near- to mid-term plans to improve the national situation holistically. In May (after the CB had been extended), the focus of JTF(A) and the Medical Intel team's efforts was to "get ahead of the curve". By this time, everyone had levelled up their knowledge of epidemiology terms and the non-medical team members were now familiar with terms such as sensitivity, specificity and PCR testing. They had also seen multiple iterations of the textbook communicable disease epidemic curve as we explored the mathematical modelling of disease transmission in the dormitories. Nationally, we were in a better state — the laboratory capacity for PCR testing had been ramped up, our serology test capability was forecasted to be operational in May, medical posts were established in all the large dormitories, and the local medical teams had established their routines and SOPs.

But each month and operational phase presented its own unique set of challenges. May's challenges were proactive ones — we had the option of serology tests. That allowed JTF(A) the ability to perform serology tests for dormitory residents who had tested positive with the PCR tests, to better understand the likely time-point at which the infection had likely occurred. At a larger scale, this allowed the operation to categorise where each dormitory was at on the epi-curve through a sample of the dormitory residents (see Fig. 2), and (b) whether infected individuals were in the early or late phase of the infection.

This was a game-changer as it gave us insights into the state of disease spread in the dormitories and on an important phenomenon (which was subsequently written up for publication) that there were significant volumes of undetected, subclinical infections in the dormitories.

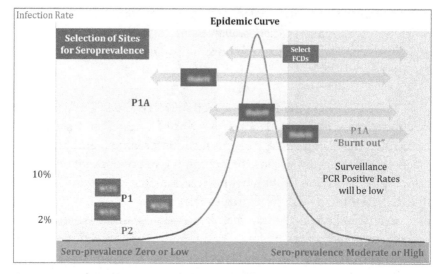

Figure 2. Illustration on how serology tests could provide insights on where each dormitory was at on the epi-curve, dated 8 May 2020.

It provided us the following insights:

(a) Ongoing transmission was more widespread and undetected than previously known;
(b) A good proportion of infections were sub-clinical and mild;
(c) Our safe distancing measures (SDMs) might not have been as effective as we thought they would be.

But it also presented new opportunities — those who were sero-positive had developed some form of immunity and protective factor, so they could return to work once the authorities were able to ascertain that they were non-infectious.

So this line of mass-testing for dormitories — using nasal swabs for PCR tests and blood tests for the serology to understand the state of each dormitory — and planning for a "return to work" and "return to normalcy" timeline for the dormitory residents continued throughout June and July.

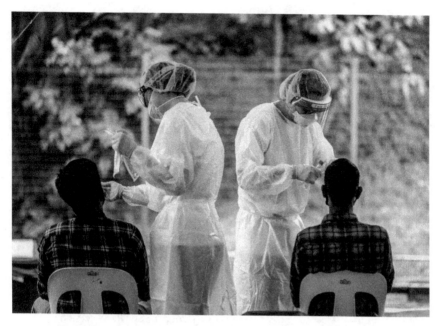

Figure 3.   Mass testing of residents using nasopharyngeal PCR swabs.
Photo credit: Alex Chua

On the sides of all these intense work, there was this huge other battle happening in the public space about (a) the high rates of infection in the dormitories and the related conversations through the medical care and human rights lens, and (b) public concerns over the high daily number of COVID-19 cases (mainly from the dormitories) as a result of these extensive proactive testing in the dormitories.

[see MOH charts In Figure 5]

The processes and protocols for the "dormitory clearance" were discussed at very high levels and fine-tuned over numerous iterations, taking into account the scientific merits and practical considerations. Broadly, the

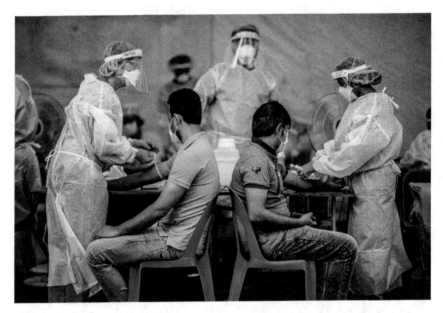

Figure 4. Mass testing of residents using blood for COVID-19 serology.
Photo credit: Alex Chua

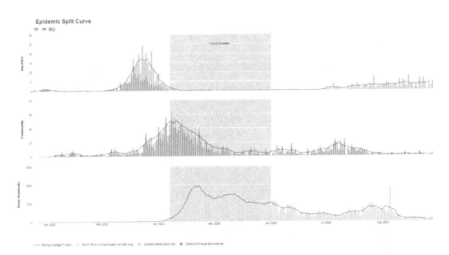

Figure 5. Epidemic curve of COVID-19 cases detected in the community and dormitory setting. Retrieved from https://covidsitrep.moh.gov.sg/, accessed on 29 August 2020.

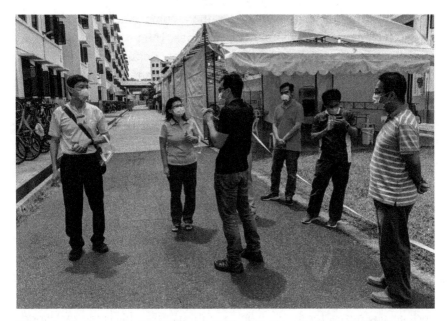

Figure 6.   Professor Leo Yee Sin and Adj A/Prof Matthias Toh from the NCID at Avery Lodge talking to the FAST team.
Photo credit: Clive Tan

plan for the lightly infected dormitories was to PCR test all the untested and uninfected residents, while for the heavily infected dormitories, everyone was to undergo serology testing. This approach was validated and assessed to be safe and operationally feasible and provided the foundation for a "return to work" and "return to normalcy" plan for the dormitory residents.

However, two issues arose mid-way through this plan: (1) Given that infections and transmission at each of the dormitories is a one-way street (i.e., they will only get more infected with time, and not less infected), the number of lightly infected dormitories dwindled as the weeks passed, and (2) there were a number of dormitories which did not fit into either of the two categories — a matter that came to be termed as the "middle of the table" issue.

It was neither timely nor ethically right to wait for these "middle of the table" dormitories to become highly infected before the residents could return to work, so a less clean-cut and more complicated process had to be created to manage this set of dormitories. The final process involved multiple and sequential testing of the dormitory population. Other than it being highly resource intensive, the process also generated by-products in the form of the high number of COVID-19 cases reported in the daily MOH reports and press releases. But the national leadership accepted this as an inevitable cost and remained steadfast in their principled and determined approach to addressing this issue "the right way".

This resulted in a surge of proactive testing in July and early parts of August, which led to the small peaks in the epidemic curve for the dormitory setting. With that, the dormitories were successfully "cleared" on 7 August, meeting the earlier promise that the Singapore government made on 24 July via its press release that all migrant worker dormitories to be cleared of coronavirus by 7 Aug.

So this chapter was successfully closed in August, and the dormitories had all been tested and cleared. Of course, we wish that the story would end happily ever after at this point, but then again, this is the real world. So it is more akin to a wildfire being smothered, but close monitoring and surveillance are still needed to watch for any resurgence or second waves, and prompt action is needed to put out these "small bushfires" before they evolve into a bigger one.

Figure 7 provides my team's recap on how our involvement and contributions evolved over the months leading up to where we were then. (See next page.)

Medical Intel and Epidemiology Team's Participation in JTF(A) – 8 April to 7 August

	April	May	June	July	August
Key Phases	Ensuring Public Order and Public Health	Getting ahead of the Transmission Curve	Restoring Public Confidence	Dorm Clearance and Return to Work	Managing Re-emergence
Partners	AOC	SPC/J5 & TOTE	SPC/J5 & TOTE	TOTE & MARIO	MARIO
			JTF Med Ops		
			MOH & RHS partners		
Key Activities	• Classify and risk-stratify Dorms • Epidemic projections • Daily COVID-19 monitoring (PBDs FCDs) • Develop Med Intel reporting dashboards for JTF • Epidemiological investigation of infection control in dorms • Investigate geographic clusters in FCDs • Prioritisation of limited testing resources	• Daily COVID-19 monitoring (PBDs FCDs) • Med Intel on plans on priorities on dorms which we can "save" • Planning for aggressive swabs to arrest escalation • Med Intel gathering on more dorms through surveillance swabs / prevalence studies • P-categorisation of dorms and movement across categories • Assist with supporting ops-research on knowledge gaps and issues pertinent to JTF operations • Exit strategy planning with SPC – differentiated testing strategy • Co-development of pooled testing protocols for JTF • Develop plans for serology	• Daily COVID-19 monitoring (PBDs FCDs) • Selection, Timing and sequencing of swab and serology ops • Partnering laboratories for results and establish effectiveness of test platforms • Development of sequential serology plans for dormitories • Scenario planning and resource planning for post-CB • Tracking new infections by site and nature of test	• Daily COVID-19 monitoring (PBDs FCDs) • Tracking new infections by site and nature of test • Co-develop SOPs with MARIO for re-emerged infections in cleared dorms • Assist JTF Med with coordination with MOH on policy matters	• Daily COVID-19 monitoring (PBDs FCDs) • Advisory services to MARIO
Team	3-man team		3-man team	Added 2 team members Worked on roster system as routine work resumes for team members	Merged into ACE

Figure 7. Overview of the phases of operation and the key activities of the Medical Intel team.

12 Personal Stories From the Frontline

NCID Doctors

Adjunct Assistant Professor Monica Chan
Senior Consultant, NCID and Head, Department of Infectious Diseases, Tan Tock Seng Hospital

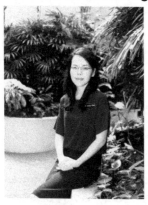

The National Centre for Infectious Diseases (NCID) has been at the forefront of the outbreak effort since the start of the outbreak when concerns of an acute febrile respiratory illness in Wuhan, China, first emerged at the end of December 2019. Outbreak plans were rapidly rolled out from early January 2020. Pre-existing working relationships between departments, both clinical and non-clinical areas, as well as various administrative committees, facilitated a whole-campus response to the fast-evolving situation. The commitment and dedication of everyone involved to provide the best possible solution in the shortest possible time were astounding. Many adaptations had to be made along the way — a number of NCID wards were opened overnight, decanting of existing patients to ward suspect cases, activation of the NCID Screening Centre within three days, the ramp-up of NCID inpatient wards capacity to house previously unimaginable numbers, infrastructure alterations to adapt wards into outbreak-ready facilities — seemingly impossible tasks during "peace-time" now became reality within days and weeks into the pandemic.

The clinicians at the NCID were ready to be first on the frontlines to provide guidance, advice and to lead by example. Despite the anxiety and uncertainty faced in those early days, we rallied together, supported each other, and faced this unprecedented crisis with a more united front than ever before. I remember the following events very clearly — receiving the first suspect case in the NCID, treating the first confirmed case in the NCID and the cases from the first local confirmed cluster, seeing the first COVID-19 ICU case, witnessing the first discharge from the hospitals and the first death at the NCID, participating in the first therapeutic trials in NCID, and many more! Each of these were memorable though it is impossible to fully describe the extent of work underlying each one.

The augmented manpower provided by the Division of Medicine medical officers, senior residents and consultants from Tan Tock Seng Hospital have been absolutely crucial to the outbreak response as inpatient numbers escalated. The camaraderie and team spirit during this crisis will remain with us as a lasting memory.

Many hours, overnights, weekends, public holidays, significant family and personal commitments have been sacrificed to ensure that our patients receive the care they needed, our staff remain protected and reassured, and the entire system works well to support Singapore's outbreak response to this pandemic. To all NCID and TTSH staff — I offer my utmost gratitude and appreciation for your commitment and dedication.

Dr Sapna Sadarangani
Consultant, NCID

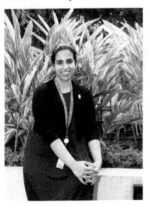

I have realised that the time scale during an outbreak with a novel pathogen is very different. It seems humanity is in the midst of an epoch in our lives. I was the ward consultant receiving suspect COVID-19 (at that time termed 2019-nCoV) patients in January 2020 and I worked in outbreak areas during the Chinese New Year long weekend when our first confirmed case and other suspect cases were admitted. I remember numerous texts and calls that weekend. I thought to myself: "Surely, the NCID Screening Centre will be activated." Indeed it was after the Chinese New Year weekend.

There have been many phases and surges during this outbreak, with numerous challenges to navigate. What has been tremendous is the teamwork and willingness of colleagues to go the extra mile, working long hours in Personal Protective Equipment (PPE) till we had marks on our faces and pressure areas on the nose bridge. We have had to be agile in modifying protocols frequently and being adaptable and flexible to change. Things evolve fast, so the dialogue between frontline clinicians and leadership is extremely crucial, as is vigilance to connect-the-dots to discover new clusters or emerging new disease manifestations.

While the experiences of senior clinicians who experienced the SARS outbreak in 2003 are invaluable, we learnt SARS-CoV-2 is a pathogen in its own right with a different viral load and disease manifestation characteristics. We had to be open to learn, understand our observations and implement changes in policy when appropriate. The efforts of research teams, nationally and globally, have been and will continue to be important, along with clinician and public health observations.

The surges from local community clusters and returning travellers in February 2020 was the beginning of the challenge on our resilience. I was touched also by the resilience of my patients. Paraphrasing the conversation with one of my patients, a young medical student who had returned from the United Kingdom: "Dr Sapna, what is the NCID's bed occupancy?... I do not feel that unwell right now and wonder if it is alright for me to be admitted instead of someone else who may need the hospital bed much more than I do..." We also had a number of family clusters and a few pregnant women affected during that time. I am grateful for colleagues from KK Women's and Children's Hospital and National University Hospital (as well as other hospitals) who we worked with to try to reunite families if parents/children were admitted into different hospitals. It was gratifying when patients expressed appreciation for our efforts to reunite them with other family members whenever feasible, during the challenging time of isolation. Caring for patients who were dying also called upon us to support patients and families through their anxiety and grief.

The outbreak in dormitories for our migrant workers was significant as it called upon public health authorities, clinicians, nurses, frontline staff, NGOs and the system to adapt and be resourceful to ensure they were well taken care of. The scale of the outbreak was not the only thing, but also the specific language and cultural considerations, and being able to support patients through psychological stress and anxiety. This has taught us that there can be gaps despite preventive measures put in place. It is good to see we made a strong attempt to bridge those gaps.

It is not only possible but important to maintain a degree of compassion amidst the busyness.

I also had the chance to speak with staff in various work areas when I initiated our healthcare worker seroepidemiological study at the NCID and Tan Tock Seng Hospital. I am thankful for their participation, and it was humbling to see the collective efforts at all areas of the campus. It truly is an all-hands-on-deck effort and everyone's contributions are important. On a personal note, although I know we have a long haul ahead of us, I am grateful for my colleagues, the health of my family, adequate PPE, efforts of public health authorities, cooperation from the community, and the things we often take for granted, e.g., each day, home, blue skies, trees, a sense of humour, and much more!

Dr Ling Li Min[1]
Visiting Infectious Diseases Senior Consultant, NCID

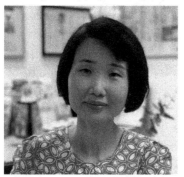

There is close, multi-disciplinary interaction in the outbreak ICUs at the NCID. We discuss with each other to gather crucial expert opinions whenever there is a clinical need. There have been many opportunities for robust discussion on patient management and sharing of literature amongst the various clinicians extending beyond the field of infectious diseases during this pandemic. It is a nice feeling knowing that one comes to work with friends, where we support each other as well as respect each other's diverse opinions.

The ICU teams have rallied through the difficult times when there were complicated patients and always gave each other moral support. There was an occasion when Dr Benjamin Ho, Director of NCID ICU, shared the photo of a newborn child of one of our patients with us. This patient was still unwell and had been in ICU for more than one month at this time. This motivated everyone to press on, and the patient eventually made it out of ICU after two and a half months.

There were also more opportunities than usual to work with many talented trainee doctors rotating through the ICU-infectious diseases team, who have shown much motivation and courage.

Good patient outcomes in outbreak ICUs illustrate that even in dire straits, miracles do happen. In every crisis, there will be many opportunities — from learning and innovation to continuously looking for ways to improve our practice for bringing out the best in people. We also learnt that it is important to prioritise activities during the day in order to maintain efficiency and that it is also necessary to have scheduled rest and time with one's family in order to recharge.

Finally, outbreak or not, we know that we need to remain current and keep ahead of the curve. We must continue to seek ways to create value for our patients, department, the institution and for our country. At the same time, we must maintain a sense of empathy towards our patients, their families and to our fellow colleagues as well.

The efficiency of the NCID machinery for managing outbreaks is nothing short of impressive. Together with the tremendous support from Tan Tock Seng Hospital (TTSH), many healthcare workers at the NCID and TTSH have been provided with a strong sense of security as they combat COVID-19. This outbreak has brought out the best in various individuals and it is both heartening and gratifying to see how everyone within public and private healthcare institutions have come together like an army to battle the outbreak.

Dr Frederico Dimatatac
Principal Resident Physician, NCID

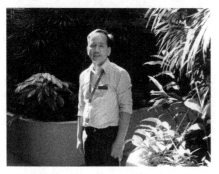

As the roster planner for Medical Officers (MOs) posted to the Communicable Disease Centre for many years and now the NCID, I typically handle around 10–12 MOs per posting. During the outbreak, roster planning became more complicated as there was now a need for daily planning, which required more time and meticulous attention to detail.

As the outbreak evolved and definitions of "suspect case" were regularly revised and updated, I had to stay updated as an increase in the number of admissions would call for me to pull the trigger and activate additional MOs for deployment to the NCID. This could mean increasing the numbers of MOs on night call from one to five, or calling up MOs in the evening to supplement the existing night call officers on duty, placing MOs on call during the weekends and public holidays, and constantly working to adjust manpower needs on the weekends.

Trust and believe in the process

As the NCID progressively opened wards to accommodate the large number of patients being admitted, more MOs were deployed. Despite having apprehensions about safety working in outbreak wards, these junior doctors were very eager and enthusiastic to help. Regular briefings with new additions were carried out by our Head of Department, Dr Monica Chan, to address concerns and to reinforce strict adherence to infection control protocols such as the donning and doffing of Personal Protective Equipment (PPE), hand hygiene, daily temperature monitoring, practising safe distancing, and the wearing of a surgical mask at all times.

We also ensured that the mental health and morale of our junior doctors were prioritised as the workload gradually increased and leaves were being cancelled. We ensured constant communication between one another to stay connected and to strengthen teamwork and camaraderie, even when we could not see our colleagues physically. I would like to give special thanks to Dr Timothy Quek, Consultant, Endocrinology, Tan Tock Seng Hospital, for his guidance and advice, and to my colleagues, for the many hours of careful planning to keep our system running well.

Dr Tay Jun Yang
Associate Consultant, NCID
"We will get through this!"

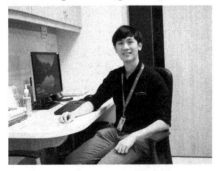

This was said during one of the first meetings in January 2020 where our department convened after work hours to discuss our strategies in containing the new unknown virus that was to be SARS-CoV-2. I remember the initial somewhat sombre tone of the meeting was immediately lifted after Dr Brenda

Ang, Senior Consultant at the NCID, pronounced that we would get through this together, as we have with SARS. The months that ensued were truly a remarkable testimony to the human spirit.

I still remember the conversation I had with my wife just prior to working in the outbreak wards at the NCID. The prospect of potentially being infected and infecting my three-month-old baby was especially daunting but my wife gave me the support I needed, adjusting our daily routines whenever required. I was fortunate to have had the support of my family as I worked on the frontlines.

Experiencing COVID-19 as a medical doctor was like fighting a long-drawn war. I had always felt that after the SARS experience in 2003, we would be more prepared for an outbreak than before — and we were. We had a war chest of scenario-planning and contingencies based upon our SARS experience. As we drew on our war chest, we had our small victorious battles, but whenever we felt that we were emerging on top, a new spanner was thrown in the works as the COVID-19 enemy was attacking us on different fronts. Within a matter of weeks, we were working on contingencies and adapting ourselves to the evolving situation. COVID-19 taught us something else — outbreaks do not conform to plans.

Yet, healthcare workers from different sectors, different specialties and different roles rose to the occasion. What I will remember for years to come is the camaraderie forged amongst those who stood at the front lines.

Nursing

Dr Margaret Soon
Director of Nursing, NCID

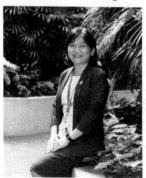

The NCID was built for 330 beds, but we were already running at half capacity when the year started. Since the NCID opened, we had been conducting training and drills for opening wards and the Screening Centre (SC). Little did we expect that the drills would be put to the test so soon.

The NCID leadership first met on 2 January 2020 to discuss the emergence of atypical pneumonia in China. Since then it has been a continuous slew of activities. Among the many things that Nursing had to do, getting the facilities ready was the foremost priority. We had to open wards and the SC, as well as decant current patients so as to convert general wards to outbreak wards. At one point, when the demand for beds was high, we started increasing capacities by cohorting two to three patients in each room.

We had prepared for all these scenarios. Immaculate planning and meticulous executions had enabled us to ready the wards with clockwork precision. However, it was how the various departments worked together in close collaboration to make things happen that left indelible memories.

I remember the day we had to prepare and open up five wards in the span of one evening. Nursing colleagues from Tan Tock Seng Hospital came over to the NCID that evening and everyone helped in whatever ways they could, from stockpiling consumables to putting up instruction posters and checking telephone lines. We had been too busy to shout out for help, but nonetheless, help came. Many departments worked past midnight that day; many going without dinner even.

It was just a few months after NCID's official opening when the outbreak started. Apart from having enough manpower to run only half the number of wards, the NCID Nursing team was also very junior, with the bulk of the workforce having been in the NCID for less than a year. In order to cope with the rapid ramp-up in the initial month, many of the nurses worked through the weekends and late into the nights without any rest days. I know of nurses who did not go home and slept in the hospital because they had worked past midnight. Many took on responsibilities way beyond their usual job scopes. For example, when the NCID Nursing Team was tasked with the mammoth task of setting up the SC and running the place for the first 72 hours, the Outbreak Team of nurses rose to the challenge and got the place going despite being just senior staff nurses (SSNs) and assistant nurse clinicians (ANCs). Everyone was stretched and visibly tired, but yet remained upbeat in all that they did.

The nurses saw it as their duty to ensure that the NCID was ready for whatever comes. I remember the evening before Chinese New Year eve, one staff member shared how she had to send her helper to buy new clothes for her children because she had not had the chance to go home before shops closed. I looked at my watch; it was almost 10.30 pm. I felt apologetic for working the nurses so hard. However, she nonchalantly replied: "Don't worry sister, my helper can do it. Others are in the same situation too," drawing the attention away from herself. I was overwhelmed with a deep sense of gratitude. These are people with spouses, children and parents. Yet, they had sacrificially and whole-heartedly given their all, worked longer hours, quietly took on additional roles with unwavering commitment and dedication.

One precious lesson I learnt in this outbreak is the importance of clear communication (even when it means honestly telling the nurses that I know just as little). There is a fine balance between communicating to raise awareness without raising alarm. At the start of the outbreak, when little was known about the disease, the staff still needed information to prepare for the inevitable impending outbreak. We conducted multiple short briefings to provide situational updates, along with infection control measures and the rationale for such measures. When we had our first positive COVID-19 test result, I remember sitting the nurses down to break the news to them first so that they could clarify any concerns they might have had. All these helped the nursing team deal with the unknown.

Ma Theresa Diamante Alandre
Senior Nurse Manager, NCID

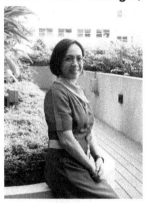

I was first involved in an outbreak training exercise earlier in 2019, where we focused on the deliberation and fine-tuning of the NCID's outbreak workflows and processes in the event of a pandemic.

Fast forward to December 2019, when we first heard the news of a novel viral pneu-monia emerging in Wuhan, China, the NCID shifted from training mode to high alert as we prepared ourselves and the facility to receive potential cases.

In the early days of the pandemic, we prepared our reserve wards to receive patients. As the number of cases started to rise, the NCID needed to increase its bed capacity. My team and I had to first transfer existing patients out of the NCID's general wards to receive confirmed COVID-19 patients. Subsequently, we had to prepare and re-purpose the wards to receive COVID-19 cases.

As the number of COVID-19 cases started to rise, NCID needed to increase bed capacity. Together with my colleagues and Nursing Leaders in the NCID and Tan Tock Seng Hospital (TTSH), we moved beds across wards and placed two or three beds into each room to double or triple the capacity of each ward.

At the height of the pandemic, the NCID was close to reaching saturation point. The nursing team then needed to prepare the identified patients to be decanted to other isolation and healthcare facilities. This required a lot of coordination with other departments to ensure a smooth transfer of patients to these facilities.

One of my tasks during this outbreak was to take care of the nurses from TTSH deployed to work in the NCID. They had to first undergo refresher training, which included donning of Personal Protective Equipment (PPE) and familiarisation of the facilities and equipment used in managing COVID-19 patients.

I was responsible for rostering the deployed nurses and assigning them to a nursing buddy. This process was a tiring and difficult one in ensuring that the right matching of skills between the staff were there. I also made sure to lend a listening ear to allay any concerns that these nurses might have while working in the NCID.

Albeit tiring, the experience I have gained in this pandemic has left an inedible mark on my psyche about managing emerging infectious diseases and outbreaks. It was also heartening to hear feedback from our staff that they feel safe while working at the NCID and to see their resilience in adapting to the constant workflow changes day in and out.

Imrana Banu
Nurse Manager, NCID

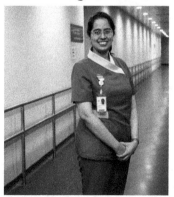

As a specialised infectious diseases clinic, we started making preparations and braced ourselves for this fight when the news about an unknown viral pneumonia outbreak in China first broke out on 2 January 2020.

During the early days of COVID-19, we had minimal information about the virus or the necessary precautions that were needed. However, well-versed with localised outbreak protocols through multiple training drills, Clinic J shifted into localised outbreak mode in order to segregate our business-as-usual (BAU) patients from the increasing number of COVID-19 suspect cases we were receiving. We closed our extended arm, the Day Treatment Centre, and put in place stringent screening and isolation protocols based on travel history and symptoms assessment for all patients. Patients who meet suspect criteria were immediately isolated in the Special Precaution Area (SPA) — a purpose-built facility with a negative pressure regime with 12 air exchanges — at Clinic J.

As the number of suspect cases to be screened increased further, it was decided that Clinic J had to scale down the volume of BAU patients cared for at the clinic. This required extensive back-end coordination with multiple stakeholders such as doctors, pharmacists and medical social workers to ensure that our BAU patients continue to receive their medications and the care they need, even if their appointments are deferred. As a certain group of patients were still required to return for follow-up care, the team was split into teams to attend to BAU patients, COVID-19 suspect cases, and any other BAU cases. With the opening of the Screening Centre (SC) in late January 2020, our clinic Patient Service Associates (PSAs) were also further deployed to the SC to train other PSAs. This led to a stretch of manpower on the ground.

On top of BAU and outbreak functions, Clinic J also supports other COVID-19-related services, such as clinical assessment of experimental therapeutic treatments, epidemiological investigations to determine possible links between cases, as well as guiding the implementation of public health measures on the ground to contain further transmission of the disease.

Workflows in the clinic were also constantly changing — by the hour, days and weeks — as a result of fast-changing recommendations, health advisories and circulars from the Ministry of Health and hospital management. Multiple meetings and reminders were needed to reinforce the changes on the ground. This involved ensuring staff compliance to infection control protocols, safe distancing measures, mask up policies and temperature monitoring, all of which were critical to ensuring both staff and patient safety.

On the patient front, we had to manage concerns from patients on their safety when returning to Clinic J for follow-up appointments and assure them that infection control practices and workflows are strictly adhered to. We also had to manage patients' fears when having to be isolated.

Two of our Clinic J staff were diagnosed with COVID-19 during the course of the pandemic. Although they were infected in the community and not during their course of work, this sparked fear amongst our staff. However, our team motivated and reassured one another with the knowledge that we all complied with the infection control measures in place and continued to do our best in our roles in ensuring both patient and staff safety.

With proper protocols and policies, and not forgetting the care and support rendered to healthcare workers, I believe we can manage COVID-19 together as one community.

Paige Phoon Long Yoke
Assistant Nurse Clinician, Outbreak Team, NCID

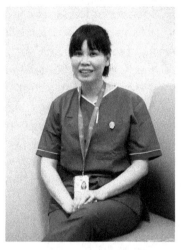

When the first suspect case of COVID-19 was reported in Singapore on 4 January 2020, my outbreak team colleagues and I were in preparation to streamline processes to manage COVID-19 in our hospital. As the largely unknown virus spread exponentially across China, fear and uncertainty began to hit me, but I knew succumbing to such feelings would render me useless and helpless. Pushing these feelings aside, I kicked myself into fight mode, working together with my colleagues to prepare everyone in facing the unknown.

In any infectious disease outbreak, the need to reinforce stringent infection control practices cannot be underestimated. Multiple infection control and mask fitting sessions were conducted in our hospital by our team. It is an unprecedented time we are facing right now, but the best part of my job as a trainer is its motivational aspects.

In sharing my infection control knowledge during these sessions and answering queries on work-place infection control practices and relevant questions about my personal experiences, I helped to allay staff anxiety. Seeing relief flood the faces of my colleagues made me feel a great sense of satisfaction.

We received multiple requests to support infection control services for external organisations as the COVID-19 outbreak progressed, inclusive of on-site walkabouts to streamline workflow, infection control training and mask fitting sessions for staff. This is when I learnt that processes are not designed to be stagnant, and there is a need to adapt accordingly to each organisation's varying clienteles and available resources. There was a need to tailor the applied flows in our hospital to ensure it is practicable and doable in each organisation without compromising the basic fundaments of infection control practices.

I have also learnt to listen and appreciate the opinions of others. People adapt better to change in work processes when the rationale of such changes is properly communicated to them. Apart from assisting them, I have had the privilege of getting to know many people from other organisations, and I look forward to working with them again in the future.

Additionally, we were tasked to train other healthcare trainers from diverse backgrounds. The questions posed by other trainers were a challenge but also created various learning opportunities for both myself and my staff. Both parties better understood the perspective of the other as we faced the uncertainty of knowledge of COVID-19.

Overall, am I satisfied and happy with my work? The answer is a definite "YES". It is a fulfilling job, and at the end of the day, I go home feeling that I have contributed to the fight against COVID-19 alongside my team members. I firmly believe that my background in infection control and pandemic training makes me the most suitable person in knowing what good preventive infection control practices to employ to ensure the safety of my colleagues, my family and myself.

Wong Yee Qing
Senior Staff Nurse, NCID

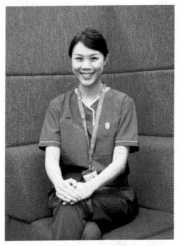

Managing patient's isolation fears

I vividly remember when a young woman (in her thirties) was admitted under my care as a suspect case for COVID-19 testing. With no presenting symptoms, she was admitted due to travel history to Bintan, Indonesia. I observed from the nurse's counter that she was sitting on the edge of the bed, appearing anxious and tense. Concerned, I decided to approach her.

Upon entering her room, she suddenly broke down into tears, saying she was "so scared". She felt imprisoned and was fearful of being alone and confined within the "four walls and a door". The inability to recognise whoever entered her room due to them being fitted in protective gear, being barred from visitors and the fear of infection and of passing the infection to her family and friends worried her. While I know that it is, unfortunately, necessary for confirmed or suspected COVID-19 patients to be isolated in rooms or wards, it is an understandable situation faced by our patients awaiting the results of their COVID-19 test.

While it sounds simple, being in isolation is more complicated than one might think. We often have to prepare these patients emotionally in the hope of decreasing their level of anxiety and helping them understand the necessity for isolation. Simple gestures such as assisting patients to connect their handphones to Wi-Fi or providing handphone chargers to help them stay connected to their families and loved ones go a long way in easing their feelings of social isolation as they remain physically isolated in the hospital. I will try to engage patients in casual conversations each time I attend to them, hoping it would give them a break from their stressful thoughts. More importantly, I always remind them that they are not alone.

Navigating Through Constantly Changing Workflows/ Recommendations

Besides focusing on the well-being of individual patients, evidence-based practice implementation is crucial in providing quality nursing care. Due to the rapidly changing nature of the COVID-19 virus, changes and adjustments in the daily workflow are necessary for coping with the pandemic.

As a frontline nurse, staying on track with constantly changing workflows and recommendations from the outbreak team and clinical specialists becomes a daily norm. Information on the latest workflows is disseminated in individual ward chats with detailed explanations at the start of each shift. At times, we observe nurses struggling to adapt to new workflows as we were not sufficiently prepared to keep up with such quick and constant changes in our daily practice. While it is often challenging to adapt to change, the on-going encouragement from our nurse managers, clinicians and colleagues was key in helping nurses navigate through the climate of constant change.

Lee Wan Lih
Senior Staff Nurse, NCID

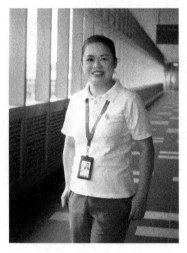

I can still recall my first intubation experience on a COVID-19 patient. Despite assisting with intubating patients in the ICU on a regular basis or having gone through regular intubation drills requiring full precautions for potential infectious cases in the NCID, I still felt a little worried when the team doctors informed us to prepare for intubating a patient. I took a brief moment to reassure myself that this would be just like any regular intubation process. As there was potential risk of human-to-human transmission, we had to don full Personal Protective Equipment (PPE) with a Powered Air-Purifying Respirator (PAPR) to ensure a higher level of protection. Heightened caution when connecting the breathing tube to the ventilator machine as we came into close contact with the patient and extra precautions, such as the use of a full set of disposable sterile requisites for the intubation process, were also taken.

Given that the NCID ICU is a fairly new facility that was only just opened a year ago, COVID-19 is the first challenge that my team of NCID colleagues and I have encountered. As per recommended protocols, we are split into two teams: one team enters the patient's room to assist with the intubation procedure while the other team observes the procedure through a CCTV to provide support from outside. To minimise the risk of infection, the headcount is capped to four in a team, whereas, previously, there would have been more manpower to assist this procedure. While the limited manpower may be challenging, we have a reliable team with all hands on deck to ensure the process goes smoothly. The supporting team ensures PPE is donned correctly and will alert the team inside to any potential breach in contamination detected through their video observation.

Another challenge that surfaced were communication difficulties due to the wearing of PPE, which hinders receiving messages through the intercom effectively. It is a potentially stressful situation if a patient's condition is deteriorating and the team inside requires more assistance.

While it is uncomfortable having to don the PPE for long hours, it gives me the confidence that I am well-protected when nursing severely ill patients, and I am not worried about having to do my job.

Jamie Lim
Deputy Director, Nursing, Tan Tock Seng Hospital

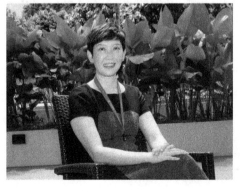

In the days leading up to my deployment to the NCID Screening Centre (SC), I was listless. I was not my usual collected self as my mind went into hyper-drive, scanning through an invisible safety checklist. Since my experience with the SARS outbreak 17 years ago, I knew I would not be able to wear my reading glasses due to the goggles and other Personal Protective Equipment (PPE). I ultimately convinced myself that the only inconvenience I would face is my presbyopia. Little did I know, I was in for another unforgettable journey and that presbyopia would be the least of my concerns.

If I were asked to describe the SC as a local cuisine, I would have to choose "Rojak" but with more complex ingredients, very much unlike what we are commonly used to. It was fascinating to work with so many family groups from the hospital, and yet with the varied sub-culture and backgrounds each group brought into SC, it presented many challenges. I can only describe the initial few weeks as a constant surge of "controlled chaos".

While I am mentally prepared to face the "virus" and know that every patient who steps into the SC could potentially carry COVID-19, the true battle lies in aiming for fluidity between teams for every shift and adapting to the frequent changes in work processes and protocols. In light of such issues, the discomfort of the PPE and fear of the virus became minor inconveniences.

After working several months in the SC, it is hard not to be overcome with an unspoken sense of kindred spirit — we eat the same bento meals, wear the same "battle gears", lament over the toilet queues, exchange beauty tips on how to protect our faces, and we even merrily fought over the last ice cream kindly donated by companies and members of the public. Just like during SARS, many new friends were made and many existing friendships were strengthened. I see communities formed and forged through hardships among the doctors, nurses, pharmacists, radiographers, allied health professionals, housekeepers, porters and security officers. The "SC Rojak" is being perfected over this battle, and the taste is becoming more palatable.

What are some of the lessons that I have learnt and some of the essential toolkits needed for a pandemic? For me, apart from the physical hardware (the building and set-ups), I think common-sense competencies (the software) are often neglected but much needed — and to have double portions of patience to work with a highly varied team. It is crucial to be highly adaptable yourself while being approachable to junior and other staff.

NCID Operations

Ignatius Ee
Manager, Executive Director's Office, NCID

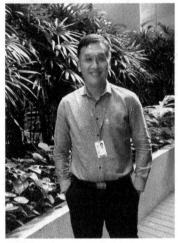

I started work at the NCID in October 2019. Having prior experience in emergency preparedness roles at Changi General Hospital (CGH) and SingHealth Polyclinics (SHP), one of my first tasks in the NCID was to support the finalisation of the NCID's Terms of Reference (TOR) during pandemic situations. My initial two months were spent engaging various stakeholders in this regard. Little did I nor the rest of the world know that dark clouds were forming on the horizon in the guise of COVID-19.

I remember going on a one-week break in early January 2020. Prior to flying off for my holiday, I returned to work on a Saturday morning to support the first COVID-19 meeting held with major stakeholders at Tan Tock Seng Hospital and the NCID. My flight was scheduled for that night. When I returned to the office a week later, the situation had taken a more urgent tone and the campus was in full swing in preparation for COVID-19. We knew that it was a matter of time before the virus reached our shores and we wanted to be prepared for it.

Multiple meetings were held to guide everyone in the same direction. I remembered coming back to the office every single day during Chinese New Year. Visits to relatives' homes and *ang baos* had to be given a miss this time around. On the third day of Chinese New Year, the decision was made to commence operations of the NCID Operations Command Centre (NOCC), which was to operate on a 24-hour, seven days a week basis. I took on the very first night shift of the NOCC and continued to work the night shifts, alternating with another colleague.

Times were indeed tough with having to alter ourselves to become nocturnal. However, we took it upon ourselves to push the envelope. As staff of the NCID, we take it upon ourselves to "be all in" in fighting this pandemic. The fight is ongoing, but we all know that we are in this together. It is an existential fight and we will triumph over COVID-19!

Jievanda Ow
Executive, Executive Director's Office, NCID

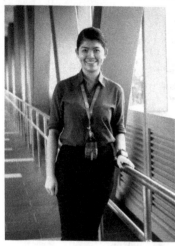

I am a fresh graduate who joined the NCID in July 2019 as a laboratory executive with the National Public Health Laboratory. As part of my job scope, I also assist the Emergency Planning — Disease Outbreak department at the NCID. A few months prior to the pandemic, we were preparing for a table top exercise and who would have known that it would come in handy so soon and that I would be battling COVID-19 in the first year of my working life.

It all started around Chinese New Year, where news was going around about the novel pathogen. I was fortunate enough to be able to celebrate Chinese New Year with my family before I was rostered to assist with operations at the NCID Operations Command Centre (NOCC). I was excited and grateful for the opportunity, but weariness kicked in as the months went on.

During the initial phase, I was rostered to work on day and night shifts. However, we were receiving increasing amounts of data that called for the need to have a dedicated team to maintain databases at the NCID. I was then assigned to a three-women-team known as the sense-making team. Our primary role focused on gathering and analysing the available data for their operational impact.

As my teammates and I are not Excel "gurus", it was laborious for us during the first few weeks maintaining and cleaning up the data. We had to plough through different data sources and trial and error with different Excel formulas in order to develop a comprehensive database. It did not end there. Due to the dynamic nature of the pandemic, we were constantly presented with new challenges, which called for us to come up with new Excel formulas as well.

On top of maintaining the database, I also assisted operations at NOCC twice a week. It is no easy feat to switch between data analysis and operations. Operation workflow and procedures change every week, and we are required to learn and adapt within the first hour or so of our operations duty. Every so often, we may find ourselves exhausted to the core at the end of the day, but we still get back up the next day to soldier on.

When it gets tough, we constantly remind ourselves that we are not alone and that if we all persist, we can fight COVID-19 to its end. As the saying goes, "When the going gets tough, the tough get going"; we persist on!

Pharmacist

Law Hwa Lin
Senior Principal Pharmacist (Specialist), NCID Pharmacy

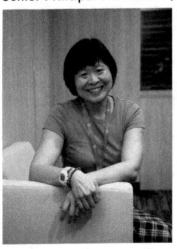

Pharmacy covers a broad range of clinical and non-clinical services. One challenge faced during a pandemic is ensuring that we have adequate resources to support outbreak response as well as balance business-as-usual (BAU) services without compromising patient care. Our Pharmacy department was split into separate teams to support COVID-19 response and BAU services. As a result of forward planning on manpower deployment and ramp-up of services, we were able to deploy staff from various sections quickly to support the NCID Screening Centre (SC) round the clock during the pandemic.

We work closely with doctors and nurses to decide on which medications to supply at the SC and on setting up standard packs of medication. In the wards, our pharmacists continue to provide medication review, medication reconciliation as well as dispensing of medications. The language barrier also became an issue with admitted patients. To prevent errors and to ensure all patients understand how to take their medications, the Pharmacy had to quickly work to produce medication labels in various languages such as Bengali, Tamil and Thai. We further shared these medication labels with other institutions, which were well-received by patients.

Although visits to the NCID's Specialist Outpatient Clinic J are scaled down, the workload at the outpatient pharmacy has not been reduced. In fact, medication delivery services have to be ramped up for patients to continue to receive their prescribed medications without visiting the hospital. Pharmacists also continue to run daily drug adherence clinics to support and ensure that our patients are adhering to their medications during these times, as well as counsel those newly started on retroviral therapy. It also serves as a platform for us to address any patient concerns related to their medications.

As COVID-19 spreads globally, securing medical and medication supplies are a further challenge faced by our procurement team. Despite earlier supply projections and negotiation with pharmaceutical companies, rationing of medications must be employed to ensure a sustainable supply chain while the team constantly looks out for medications that can be re-purposed. Pharmacists also work with physicians on the research of therapeutic treatment for COVID-19 patients, writing therapeutic guidelines on re-purposed medications as well as submitting papers for publication.

During a pandemic, we realise the importance of collective leadership. I believe that it is not possible for any leader to command operations without support from his or her staff. With this collective leadership mentality, everyone rose up to the occasion to do what needs to be done. It is also important to keep an open mind to adapt quickly to changes, think ahead, and communicate with staff constantly. Open communication allays fears and concerns that staff could have in order to support this outbreak response. Lastly, I believe that resilience, through staying physically and mentally healthy, would be key to winning this marathon against COVID-19.

Medical Social Worker

Dr Ho Lai Peng
Senior Principal Medical Social Worker, NCID

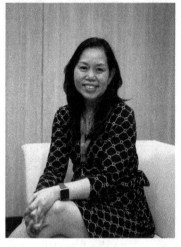

COVID-19 has undeniably challenged the way we do things. Right from the beginning, we had to re-imagine and redefine the ways to do our work. The situation was quickly unravelling and evolving, and there were a lot of uncertainties that we had to constantly adjust to.

Early on in the outbreak, the Medical Social Work team decided to split into two teams — one team to see business-as-usual (BAU) cases and the other team to see COVID-19 patients in the wards. When the alert level was raised to DORSCON Orange, we further split the teams — one team re-located to Tan Tock Seng Hospital to see BAU inpatients from the NCID, one team continued to see BAU outpatients at the NCID, and the last team to see COVID-19 patients in the NCID wards. We not only split our work but segregated the teams because there was a real fear that any one of us could be infected and our whole team could be down. It was hard to be segregated where there is no physical support from colleagues in the office that we are used to.

As most outpatient appointments were postponed, we reviewed patients over the phone. In a profession where social support to our patients is an essential part of our work, we had to find ways to maintain connection with them, which we did through phone calls or text messages and e-mails. It was not just a matter of us providing support to them; our patients sent us encouraging messages as well. I was particularly worried about a patient who was once chronically depressed and had expressed suicidal ideation. However, the pandemic caused him to rethink his life and to slowly let go of the burden of his past relationships. When he eventually let go his burdens, his emotional pain was greatly reduced and he was able to move on with his life. I am glad that something positive came out of this pandemic for him.

For the team managing COVID-19 patients, we were initially unsure about our role in the pandemic. Patients were feeling distressed by the long periods of isolation and being away from their families, especially patients in the ICU with family members who might be in quarantine. We helped to connect them to their family members through video calls or voice messages. We also addressed their feelings of fear, anger, frustration and sadness. Grief work is always difficult, but it becomes even more so when family members cannot be by the side of their family member who is dying. We help to facilitate the process of grieving by helping them find expression for their pain and make sense of their experience. This crisis has made me realise that none of us are spared from this, but it has taught me that crises could be a time of learning and reflection for all of us. I have also come to realise in our segregation from the rest of the world, how interdependent we all are. We are in this together and we can only get out of this pandemic if we help one another, especially the people and countries who are more vulnerable. We are not alright until everyone is alright.

National Public Health and Epidemiology Unit, NCID

Epidemiology and Data Sensing Team[2]

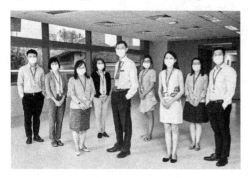

With the pandemic unfolding from China to the rest of Asia and the world, we monitor the daily incidence and mortality numbers, and highlight to our frontline colleagues to look out for potential imported cases.

As more cases emerge locally, we collect information about local clusters, study epidemiologic risk factors, and identify factors to prevent and control COVID-19 infection.

There is an immense amount of literature locally and internationally. Another role we have as the epidemiological team at the NCID is to screen through and decide which are scientifically relevant or meaningful to share with our clinicians and management team to support the fight against the pandemic.

In April 2020, the number of locally-acquired cases in Singapore ballooned rapidly. As we dealt with the fast-rising numbers daily, we needed to think out-of-the-box to scale up "out-of-hospital" facilities to house recovering COVID-19 cases who are well but not able to be discharged yet because of prolonged shedding of the SARS-CoV-2 virus. Our team had to work very quickly to identify patients who will likely remain well in a community care setting and others at higher risk who may require additional or intensive care in an acute hospital. After several rounds of analysis and deliberation with our clinicians, we finally found some meaningful patterns and recommended segregation of care to fit people of different care needs. Our analysis then helped colleagues in the Ministry of Health to drive the development of Community Isolation Facilities (CIFs).

While we project trends based on observed data of our patients and use these as norms for planning healthcare resources, our team is cognisant that there will be exceptions and outliers. A small handful of patients return from Community Recovery Facilities (CRFs) to the NCID for mild problems and often unrelated to COVID-19 infection. We continue to monitor trends after the implementation of our recommendations and are prepared to adjust the criteria if the situation changes.

With the rapidly evolving situation locally and globally, we often have to adjust and adapt along the way and respond within tight timelines. Due to the lack of data and/or little information, especially during the initial phase of the COVID-19 pandemic, we had to spend more time on the compilation of information from multiple sources. Having a resilient team and effective collaboration are essential for coping with the demands of our work.

National Public Health Laboratory Medical Technologists

Loh Pei Ling
Senior Medical Technologist, National Public Health Laboratory, NCID

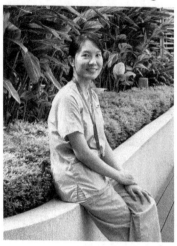

As a Medical Technologist for the past 20 years, testing rows of samples placed in front of me was my job and responsibility, but to me, they were lifeless test tubes.

These test tubes suddenly had special meaning in my life when I realised that the COVID-19 samples mean so much to patients and their anxious family members who are waiting for the results. I was one such anxious family member when I learnt that my husband tested positive in the early stages of the pandemic. Everything happened very quickly; within a day he was tested positive at the NCID, and separated from me and our children for more than 20 days. I will never forget the period when he was isolated in the NCID, and the kids and I were warded in KK Women's and Children's Hospital. I remember waiting helplessly and anxiously for daily updates on our results, always hoping to get a negative test result.

There are thousands of families out there experiencing what I had gone through — waiting for the day when their loved ones are tested negative and discharged. The faster we test samples and the test results come out negative, it means, the faster families are reunited again.

This has made me appreciate my job even more now, realising that behind each test sample and its result, there is special meaning and a direct impact on many lives and families.

Samantha Ooi
Medical Technologist, National Public Health Laboratory, NCID

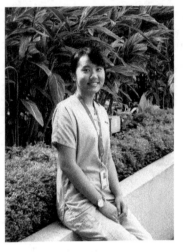

Never did I expect my first job upon graduating to be one where I am one of the frontliners in the fight against a global pandemic. Just as I was settling in and completed my probation, the first local COVID-19 case was reported in Singapore. Soon after, the number of local cases reported daily increased and adjustments had to be made to our work.

When I was told that we had to shift from our routine work to focus on COVID-19 testing, it seemed daunting as I did not know what to expect in the upcoming months. My worst fear was bringing the virus home to my parents. I was one of the newest additions to the team, and there was a lot of learning on the job and adapting to different situations as the pandemic progressed. It definitely gets stressful when your workload increases and hundreds of samples are waiting to be tested. That means having to work faster while still being 101% focused on the job and ensuring the safety of not only yourself but your team members too. Thankfully, I have very patient and supportive colleagues who made this transition easier with their guidance. It has no doubt been challenging but it has also been a rewarding experience that has allowed me to learn so much in such a short time.

Looking ahead, I hope for the world to recover from this pandemic and for life to return to normal as much as possible. I am also looking forward to being able to gather with family and friends again. I hope the experience gained during the COVID-19 pandemic has better prepared us for the future.

Healthcare Workers Who Had COVID-19*

Pauline Yue
Patient Service Associate, NCID

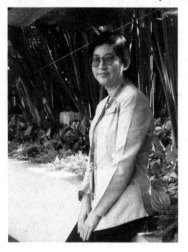

When I first found out I tested positive for COVID-19, I felt very shocked and was in disbelief. Although this virus is all we have been hearing about or dealing with every day, it never crossed my mind that this would happen to me and it felt unreal. Moreover, I did not present with symptoms and was well prior to running a fever. I am still bewildered as to where or how I was infected. I tried to recall my work assignments to explore any possibilities that I was infected during my course of work. However, I was certain I had taken all the necessary preventive measures and this possibility was quickly refuted. I remember feeling worried and guilty as I did my best to recall those that I came in close contact with before I developed a fever. I had anxiously started texting these people and advised them to avoid meeting anyone for the time being and to monitor their own health while expressing my apologies at the same time. As I nervously waited for the ambulance to pick me up, I kept feeling as if I needed to get away from everyone as soon as possible. Although I had a lot on my mind, I wasn't worried about my own health and safety as I am confident of Singapore's healthcare system and our healthcare teams, and that I would be well taken care of at the NCID.

Liew Wei Qin
Staff Nurse, NCID

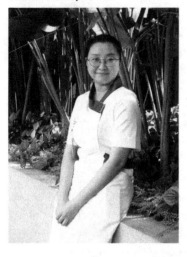

I never thought that one day I would be one of the confirmed cases. After my second swab, I thought I would receive a call informing me that I tested negative, just like the same as with my first swab result. Life, however, is full of the unexpected. I got a call from one of the doctors from the NCID, who told me I had tested positive. The first thing that went through my mind was if I had accidentally spread the virus to other people. I worried about my colleagues, my housemates, and also members of the public.

I started to worry about how to inform my parents, as I did not want them to worry about me. I did not worry much about myself as I was only experiencing mild symptoms and I believed that NCID healthcare professionals would take good care of me during my admission. However, as I had recently joined the NCID, I felt like a burden who had created trouble for my colleagues. I worried about whether it would affect my work, as I wanted to fight this war against the virus with my colleagues as well. Eventually, I knew I should focus on getting better quickly instead of worrying. I am thankful to my colleagues and friends who went out of their way to provide me emotional support and made sure I did not feel like a burden. I am also thankful to all the healthcare professionals who cared for me during this difficult time.

*Both healthcare workers were infected in the community. While carrying out their duties, they were in Personal Protective Equipment (PPE) and had observed all safe management measures. There was no onward transmission during the course of their care duties.

Support Service Staff

Chuah Swan It[3]
Senior Security Officer, Tan Tock Seng Hospital

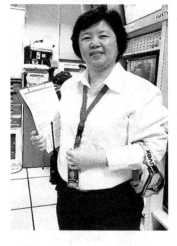

I have worked with Tan Tock Seng Hospital (TTSH) for the past two and a half years and am the mother of two children in primary and secondary school.

Before the pandemic, my duties include patrolling the campus to ensure the buildings are secure, responding to reports on suspicious objects, and access control duties. Other duties include quick responses to incidents in the clinics/wards and crowd control management. My responsibility as Senior Security Officer is to ensure the safety and security of the hospital environment for staff, patients and visitors.

Our job scope has expanded in three significant ways since the start of the outbreak. Firstly, we are required to be fitted in full Personal Protective Equipment (PPE) at designated deployment locations, e.g., the NCID Screening Centre (SC). Secondly, we are responsible for ensuring all staff are appropriately fitted in full PPE before entering any location deemed as high risk. We ensure no unauthorised individual enters the SC, and patients exiting the SC must be cleared by the SC staff. We also oversee the travel and health declarations from vendors/contractors entering the loading bays.

Finally, Security supports the transfer and escort of COVID-19 patients. These transfers include decanting of clinically stable patients to community isolation facilities as well as those who require intra-campus transfers for ongoing treatment (X-Ray, scans, etc.). Our duty is to ensure the safety of any/all unprotected individuals along these patient transfer routes.

As the news reports began emerging out of Wuhan in January 2020 with little still known of the virus, I was very nervous. Being a member of the security team at TTSH and the NCID, I understood we would be on the frontlines of Singapore's fight against the virus and our job scopes would be deeply affected. I consciously stepped up on my own personal hygiene practices. Even though my family members were worried for me, they were supportive in encouraging me to give my best at work while advising me to practice more caution.

Adjusting to being fitted in full PPE for prolonged periods of time was a challenge. Although I knew it was very important for my own safety, the difficulty of breathing in the N95 mask, the fogging up of our goggles during duty, and the added humidity of the water-impermeable gown made the experience quite uncomfortable. Being fitted in full PPE while transporting patients was even more challenging. Gradually, I adapted, and many months later, I am now more comfortable in full PPE.

Other challenges faced were keeping up to date on all patient transfer routes and infection control guidelines. I am thankful for the constant reminders, support and guidance of my Team Leaders and Supervisor. Their dedication and the team's collective effort made adjusting to these constant changes a lot easier.

Ramakrishnan Nadarajah[4]
Assistant Contract Manager, ISS Facility Services

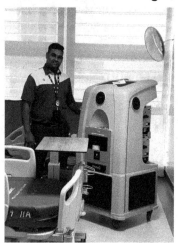

I joined ISS Facility Services Pte Ltd in 2002 and was part of the housekeeping team in Tan Tock Seng Hospital (TTSH) that fought against SARS. I left ISS in 2012, but when I re-joined in 2013, I was deployed to TTSH and have been at the NCID since it opened.

Before COVID-19, many of my colleagues have never handled an outbreak before. Our closest reference to handling an outbreak was in emergency preparedness exercises, for example, exercises in Ebola outbreak preparedness. In these exercises, we were required to don additional Personal Protective Equipment (PPE) such as googles and hairnets.

With the COVID-19 outbreak, the standard protocol for cleaning isolation rooms is to wear an N95 mask, gown and gloves when we enter the wards to do the cleaning and disinfecting of patients' rooms.

I am trained and certified to operate HPV (Hydrogen Peroxide Vapouriser) machines to disinfect isolation rooms. HPV machines dispense hydrogen peroxide in vapour form to disinfect the entire isolation room. All rooms must be sealed before operating the HPV machine. The training sessions have been an integral part of our fight against COVID-19.

Even though we have been trained in simulated outbreak scenarios to be mentally prepared for an emergency, facing a real outbreak will inevitably cause some anxiety. As the virus was unknown in the initial stages, we were concerned but allayed our fears by keeping abreast of new developments through group chats and adhering strictly to infection control protocols.

As the DORSCON level changed to Orange, major changes were made. All staff were required to do temperature checks twice a day and reminded to practise good hand hygiene.

More stringent measures were put in place with the onset of the circuit breaker. As a Malaysian, travel restrictions meant I could not return home. However, we were well-provided for in terms of our accommodation and food. Even though I cannot be with my family, ISS provided hotel rooms for us in close proximity to TTSH and the NCID to ensure that we are well-rested.

As the number of positive cases surged, so did the number of terminal cleaning cases. Wearing the PPE for long hours at times can be stressful. It was very challenging for our staff, especially those deployed to the NCID Screening Centre and COVID-19 wards. We completed multiple terminal and step-up cleanings during our 12-hour shift. Although it was quite tiring at times, we felt compelled to give our best. Through teamwork, we managed to overcome the odds.

The fear of this unknown virus is there. It has claimed thousands of lives worldwide, but we are determined to carry out our duty. We believe that we can defeat this disease. Our training in infection control has prepared us and instilled confidence in facing up to the challenge.

Our job requires us to contain the spread of the virus for the safety of all parties. At the same time, we have to take care of our family. My main goal is to ensure constant vigilance, practise good hand hygiene, and strictly follow infection control protocol so that we will be safe.

None of this would have been possible without the support of the hospital management team, ISS and the doctors, nurses, and all other hospital staff. I am touched by the community's show of care and concern in their appreciative gestures towards all frontline staff; from contributing food and drinks to notes of gratitude and care packs. A simple "thank you" meant a lot to us and made our day.

Lastly, we hope things will improve so that my colleagues, other hospital staff and I can be with our family again.

ECMO Team Members Deployed to NCID

Rosemarie Low[5]
Perfusionist, National Heart Centre Singapore

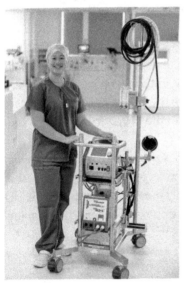

I volunteered to be part of the NCID ECMO (extracorporeal membrane oxygenation) team without any expectations or idea on what or how it would be like. I felt a little unsure in the new environment on my first activation in the NCID in March 2020. In the new state-of-the-art facility, there was a steep learning curve and I had to quickly learn the building layout while staying mindful of the strict Personal Protective Equipment (PPE) standards and disinfection protocols in place that work to minimise the chances for cross-contamination and provide self-protection.

What first started out as uncertain footing, quickly morphed into a valuable experience of working cohesively with other healthcare professionals from various institutions and backgrounds, who were deployed to the NCID for a common purpose — to provide the best standard of care for the critically ill. It was truly a joy to work with such a diverse, welcoming and knowledgeable team.

As we were doing 12-hour shifts without off days, I made sure to get adequate rest and nice home-cooked meals (*thanks mum!*) in between my shifts. I also attempted to squeeze in a yoga session or brisk walk with my dog when possible, to relax and make the most of my hours spent outside of work.

I had the opportunity to work with the NCID ECMO team again in April and May 2020 and attribute my memorable experiences in the NCID to first the people, followed by the food. When we were first orientated by the Senior Executive (*who deserves a special mention as she went to great lengths to take great care of us during our deployment there each time; thank you, Pui Yoke!*) in March, the makeshift pantry was sparse. But when I was deployed there again, there were new varieties of drinks, snacks, different flavours of cup noodles as well as vitamin C tablets and bottles of essence of chicken! The NCID had received donations from companies and members of the public to motivate us to get through the pandemic on the frontlines.

I quickly made friends over catered Bentos, where I could listen to stories from people from other healthcare institutions. Also, as not everyone was familiar with ECMO, we had impromptu sharing sessions and discussions over meals and along corridors as well. Strangers turned into acquaintances, who then turned into friends.

Some lessons learnt:

1. With a common goal and unanimous teamwork, everyone is a newfound ally and camaraderie will prevail
2. Make sure to follow all the PPE and decontamination protocol — there are posters properly thought out and nicely illustrated, and displayed at eye level all around the wards, as a reminder for all.
3. Take the initiative to read up on things that are new to you or delve deeper into your own speciality, so that when anyone comes to you with questions, you are well-prepared.

Working on the frontlines during an outbreak has not changed my view of work but has instead reinforced why I do what I do and heightened my passion and purpose towards the perfusion practice.

Angalaprameswary D/O Paniersalavam[6]
Senior Staff Nurse, Singapore General Hospital

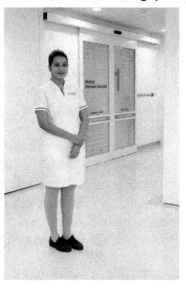

Before the first COVID-19 case arrived in Singapore, we were already briefed by our supervisors on the approach and workflows to abide by when managing such cases. We also conducted drills to ensure that everyone in the team knew what to do. As things were pretty uncertain then, I had to mentally prepare myself for the unexpected so that I could contribute effectively as a team member.

I am an ECMO-trained nurse, working in Singapore General Hospital's Medical Intensive Care Unit. Because of my training, I was informed in February 2020 that I would be deployed to the National Centre for Infectious Diseases (NCID) along with two other nursing colleagues to care for very ill COVID-19 patients who needed to be placed on EMCO.

ECMO, or extracorporeal membrane oxygenation, adopts the heart and lungs functions of patients with severe respiratory failure. However, it may cause thrombosis (blood clots) and bleeding which could be life-threatening for patients. We therefore had to monitor them closely and troubleshoot the ECMO machine when necessary to avoid adverse events. Adapting swiftly to changing conditions of the patients was a challenge but definitely an eye-opening experience.

We also had to assist in transporting COVID-19 ECMO patients for their Computed Tomography (CT) scans which required a comprehensive effort by ECMO physicians, intensivists, nurses, perfusionists and allied health staff. CT scans aid doctors in diagnosing and/or evaluating their medical treatment plans. The scans usually take no more than 15 minutes.

However, as meticulous care and attention was required to ensure the safety of patients and fellow colleagues, the entire process took more time.

Working alongside with NCID nurses for a period of six to seven months from April to November 2020 has broadened my nursing experience as we had many opportunities to learn from each other. The experiences I had will stay with me for a long time.

Photo Acknowledgments:

1. Photo credit: Dr Ling Li Min
2. Photo credit: National Centre for Infectious Diseases
3. Photo credit: Benjamin Wong, Tan Tock Seng Hospital
4. Photo credit: Sim Chin Seng, ISS Facility Services
5. Photo credit: National Heart Centre Singapore
6. Photo credit: Singapore General Hospital

Our appreciation to Henry Lim from Tan Tock Seng Hospital Communications who contributed the rest of the photos of the staff in this chapter.

Index

CPSIA information can be obtained
at www.ICGtesting.com
Printed in the USA
JSHW050445290522
26333JS00005B/89